PROSTATE BIOPSY

Edited by **Nabil Kaddis Bissada**

Prostate Biopsy
Edited by Nabil Kaddis Bissada

Published by InTech
Janeza Trdine 9, 51000 Rijeka, Croatia

Publishing Process Manager Daria Nahtigal

Technical Editor Teodora Smiljanic

Cover Designer InTech Design Team

Additional hard copies can be obtained from orders@intechopen.com

Prostate Biopsy, Edited by Nabil Kaddis Bissada
p. cm.
ISBN 978-953-307-702-4

For EU product safety concerns:
IN TECH d.o.o., Prolaz Marije Krucifikse Kozulić 3, 51000 Rijeka, Croatia,
info@intechopen.com or visit our website at intechopen.com.

Meet the editor

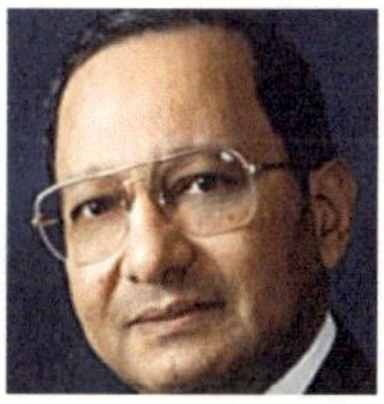

Dr. Nabil K. Bissada helds position of Professor and program Director in the Department of Urology at University of Arkansas for Medical Sciences, where he is also an Executive Vice Chairman. Among numerous important positions Dr. Bissada is also a President of Arkansas Urological Society. With the reputation as a master surgeon, his operative techniques are widely quoted. In his career, Dr. Bissada treated patients in 5 continents. He published 21 books and book chapters and authored over 300 publications.

Contents

Preface

Prostate cancer is the most common non-skin cancer, accounting for one third of all visceral cancers and the second leading cause of cancer-related death for men in the United States and is a very common cancer in developed nations. Prostate cancer incidence rates rose in the 1980s, reflecting improvement in detection and diagnosis through the widespread use of PSA. The trend in death rates in prostate cancer increased in the 1970s and 1980s then declined in the last decades. This may reflect a wider use of radical prostatectomy in localized prostate cancer especially with better understanding of the anatomical locations of the neurovascular bundles. Likewise, the reduction of reported incontinence and erectile dysfunction after radical prostatectomy in recent studies as well as the advancements in radiotherapy for prostate cancer may have contributed to this observed decline. Another possible explanation is the increased early detection of prostate cancer following the introduction of PSA screening. Whether this reduction is related to PSA screening or not will continue to be a subject of intense debate.

Prostate biopsy is the definitive modality in diagnosing prostate cancer. Numerous publications have addressed prostate biopsy in the last several decades. The crucial need for addressing the various aspects of prostate biopsy in a comprehensive volume remained unanswered until now. I hope that this book authored by many recognized world authorities in prostate cancer will provide this crucial need.

Professor Nabil Kaddis Bissada
Department of Urology
University of Arkansas for Medical Sciences
USA

1

The Development of the Modern Prostate Biopsy

Lehana Yeo, Dharmesh Patel, Christian Bach, Athanasios Papatsoris, Noor Buchholz, Islam Junaid and Junaid Masood
Barts and the London NHS Trust
UK

1. Introduction

In the 1950s prostate cancer was known to occur in about 20% of men over the age of 55 and was the cause of death in about 5% of white men over the age of 50 (Huggins and Johnson, 1947). It accounted for 90% of all male genital cancers and 63% of male genitourinary cancers and it was believed that 5-10% of prostatic cancers were diagnosed early enough to permit operation with a reasonable chance of cure (Kaufman et al., 1954). Clearly diagnosis was paramount in order to initiate treatment and improve prognosis.

The current accepted practice of diagnosing prostate cancer relies on histopathological examination of prostatic tissue obtained through transrectal ultrasound (TRUS) guided biopsy of the gland (Heidenreich et al, 2010). The TRUS-guided transrectal method of obtaining prostatic tissue has been described since the mid-1980s but before then, other methods of sampling the prostate gland were used.

This chapter describes the development of the modern prostate biopsy from the techniques of the early 1900s of transperineal open biopsy to the current method of using ultrasound guidance to allow transrectal prostate biopsies.

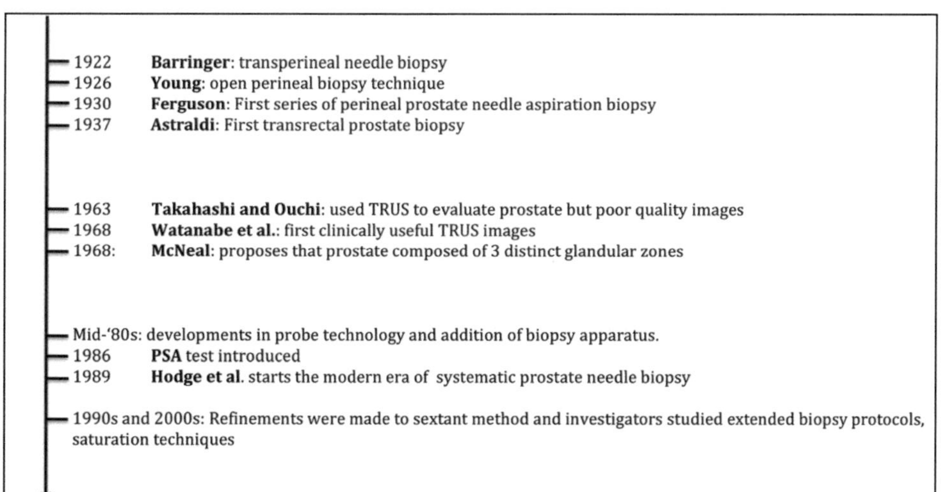

Fig. 1. A timeline of the development of the modern prostate biopsy

2. Digital rectal examination

Prior to the development of prostate ultrasound imaging the only method available to examine the prostate was by the subjective digital examination of the anterior rectal wall. Any nodularity, firmness or irregularity of the prostate raised the suspicion of prostate cancer (figure 2).

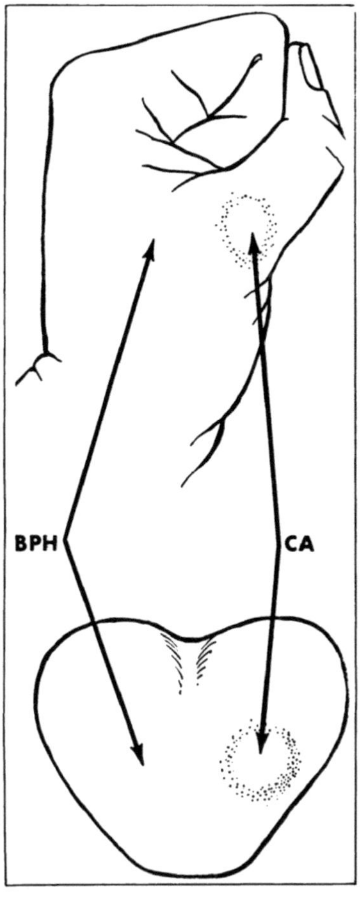

Fig. 2. Any hard lump of prostate was considered indicative of cancer unless proven otherwise (Grabstald, 1965a; Kaufman et al., 1954)

These findings along with a freely mobile prostate, normal serum acid phosphatase and normal skeletal radiographs suggested organ-confined disease and provided enough evidence to initiate radical treatment.

In 1953, Colby retrospectively reviewed 100 prostatectomy specimens for presumed prostate cancer and of these 42 were performed solely on the basis of an abnormal digital rectal examination (DRE) (Colby 1953). He found that without a histological diagnosis the surgeon correctly diagnosed cancer only 58% of the time consequently 42% of patients had had prostatectomy for benign disease. He concluded that "it seems unwise to embark upon radical surgery of the prostate without definite histological evidence of cancer". Clearly over diagnosis of prostate cancer was a significant problem and therefore it was important for the physician to obtain prostate biopsies for tissue diagnosis if there was any suspicion of prostate cancer, and certainly prior to any planned radical surgery or indeed surgical castration by way of orchidectomy.

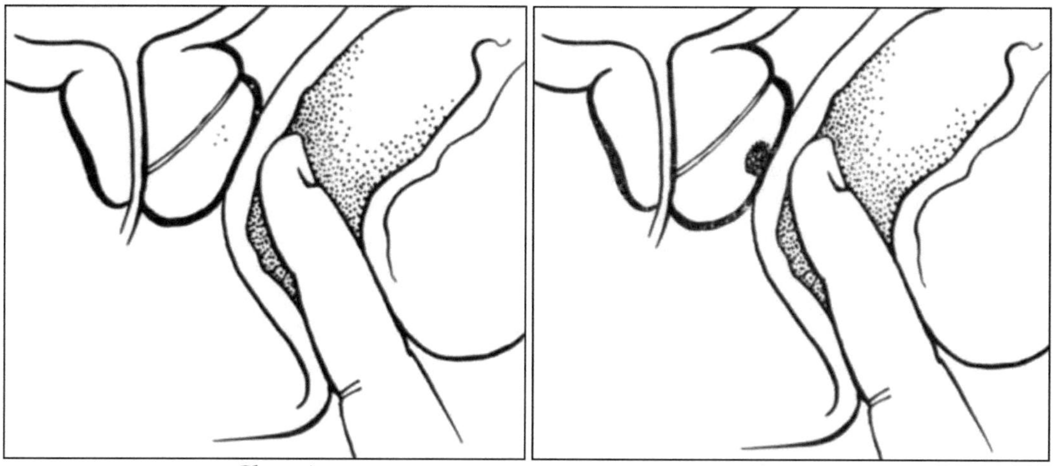

Class A Class B

Fig. 3. The early clinical classification of prostate based on digital rectal examination.

Class A (Latent): occult cancer and normal DRE, diagnosis is usually made following surgical removal for supposedly benign prostatic hypertrophy; class B (Early): an isolated small nodule is palpated within the prostatic capsule and has not metastasized (Grabstald, 1965c)

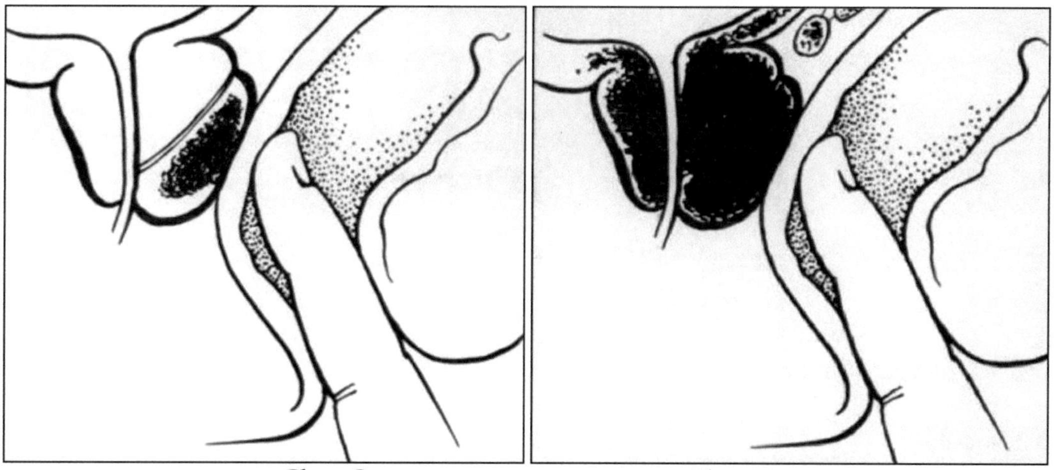

Class C Class D

Fig. 4. The early clinical classification of prostate based on digital rectal examination.

Class C (Advanced): locally extensive and may involve one or both lobes, but has not metastasized; class D (Metastases): usually similar to class C but has metastasized (Grabstald, 1965c)

3. Transperineal biopsy

3.1 Open

The earliest method of collecting prostatic tissue was by open perineal biopsy and this was once considered the most accurate technique available to detect prostate cancer. The method was mainly used in patients who were subsequently likely to require curative prostatectomy.

The procedure described by Young involved a transverse incision between the ischial tuberosities 2 cm above the anus (Young, 1926). The ischiorectal fossa was then opened by blunt finger dissection, carrying the dissection medially and reflecting the rectum posteriorly. The central tendon of the perineum was then cut exposing the recto-urethralis muscle which was opened by sharp dissection and reflected laterally, exposing the capsule of the prostate (figure 5). The abnormal area on the prostate was grasped with Allis forceps and excised widely and deeply. The cut edges of the prostate were then brought together with sutures.

Reports suggested frozen-section diagnoses should be more than 95% accurate although the risks of incontinence and erectile dysfunction were present. Consequently it was not a technique to be used in any numbers and also required a general anaesthetic and a week of hospitalization (Peirson and Nickerson, 1943).

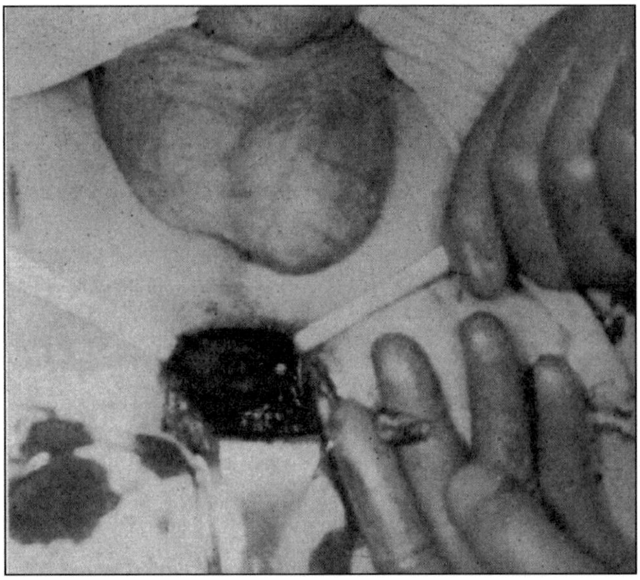

Fig. 5. Open perineal biopsy of prostate with the prostate exposed (Kaufman et al., 1954).

3.2 Needle

A technique that carried less risk and could be performed as an office procedure was the method of needle biopsy of the prostate through the perineum. The first description came in 1922 from Barringer who adopted Martin and Ellis' technique of needle puncture for acquiring tissue for histological analysis (Barringer, 1922). He described the use of a screw tip needle to obtain a perineal punch biopsy and was successful in obtaining prostatic tissue in 16 out of 33 patients.

In 1930 Ferguson modified the technique and published his series of 280 patients who had prostate needle aspiration biopsy using an 18-gauge needle via the transperineal approach and was able to remove adequate tissue in 78 to 86% of his cases (Ferguson, 1930) (figure 6). The patient was placed in the lithotomy position and local anaesthetic was infiltrated just lateral to the median raphe 1cm anterior to the anus. The index finger of the left hand was introduced into the rectum guiding an 18 gauge needle introduced into the perineum taking care to avoid the rectum and urethra. As the needle reached the prostatic capsule the plunger attached to the needle was drawn out creating a high vacuum system and simultaneously the needle was advanced through the abnormal nodule. This resulted in a small plug of tissue sharply cut within the needle. In order to cut off the tissue the needle was withdrawn 0.5-1 cm and advanced at a different angle ensuring negative pressure was maintained on the plunger whilst the needle was withdrawn to the prostatic capsule and only then the plunger was slowly released and disconnected from the needle. The biopsy needle was the quickly removed from the perineum and the tissue in the needle expressed onto a slide by re-inserting the obturator through the needle.

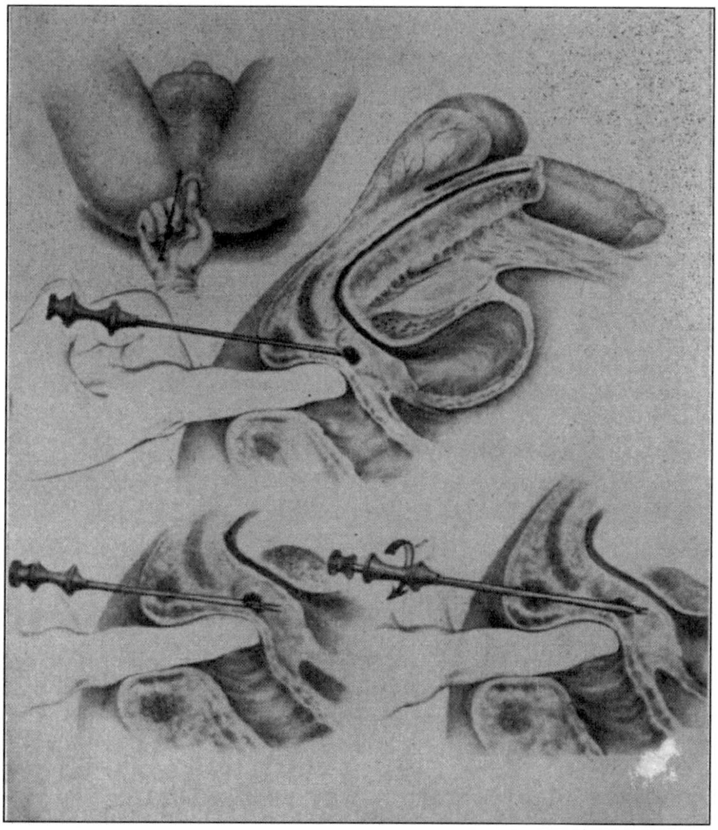

Fig. 6. Transperineal needle biopsy of the prostate (Kaufman et al., 1954)

With regards to needle aspiration, Peirson and Nickerson argued that the punch technique was more useful since in their experience it was not always possible to obtain sufficient tissue via needle aspiration and furthermore the tissue obtained amounted to a smear of

cells on the slide with loss of architecture thus making diagnosis difficult (Peirson and Nickerson, 1943). Barringer also commented that they could detect prostate cancer early only 50% of the time by aspiration biopsy (Barringer 1942).
Enthusiasm for needle prostate biopsy dwindled during the 1940s as a number of negative articles were published by prominent urologists. One report described two patients who had negative prostate biopsies and later developed advanced prostate cancer (Boyd and Nuckells, 1940).
Unfortunately not much more was published about prostate aspiration biopsies for the next 20 years. Then in 1960 Parry and Finelli described a modified method which was highly successful in allowing a directed biopsy through the perineum (Parry and Finelli, 1960). Their technique afforded greater needle control by using digital-guidance. The needle was introduced 1cm above the anus just to the right of the midline depending on the location of the lesion and with a finger in the rectum the surgeon follows the needle point along its entire course form within the anal sphincter to the prostatic nodule allowing the prostate to be stabilized in contrast to the later described method of transrectal digital guided biopsy where the nodule tended to get pushed away from the needle. Kaufman et al. also used the same technique (figure 6) and recommended that if the biopsy was benign the test could be repeated or the urologist could even proceed to open perineal exposure (figure 5) to take more histological material (Kaufman et al., 1954).
Certainly as the techniques and expertise improved reports suggested an overall 88% rate of accuracy when used to obtain tissue from a suspicious area in the prostate. Furthermore advantages were that the tissue could be studied on permanent rather than on frozen sections and repeat biopsy was easily accomplished, local anaesthetic was generally sufficient, there were little risks of erectile dysfunction, rectal injury or incontinence (Grabstald, 1965b) and it was believed that the possibility of causing seeding along the needle tract was remote (Kaufman et al., 1954).

4. Transurethral biopsy

Transurethral biopsy of the prostate was another approach that had been described but unlike the previous method described it required a general anaesthetic and a period of hospitalization. Denton et al. held that an extensive transurethral prostatectomy would nearly always confirm the diagnosis (Denton et al., 1967) and Grabstald commented that this transurethral biopsy might be useful in advanced tumours (Grabstald, 1965b).
However it was well known that prostate cancer was more frequently seen posteriorly and near the capsule and thus was not easily reached with the resecting loop since only the tissue within the prostatic urethra was sampled (Peirson and Nickerson, 1943; Kaufman et al., 1954). In a series published by Peirson and Nickerson, one patient had 4 grams of tissue resected for histology during transurethral prostate biopsy and this was later found to be benign. However since DRE was suspicious for cancer a perineal punch biopsy with the Silverman needle was performed and this subsequently revealed malignancy (figure 7) (Peirson and Nickerson, 1943). Consequently Kaufman et al. held that the procedure should not be performed as a primary biopsy technique but it may be useful to perform transurethral resection in those symptomatic of obstructive urinary symptoms (Kaufman et al., 1954). Indeed Purser et al. found that tissue taken via needle biopsy was more reliable than a limited specimen obtained via the urethra (Purser et al, 1967).

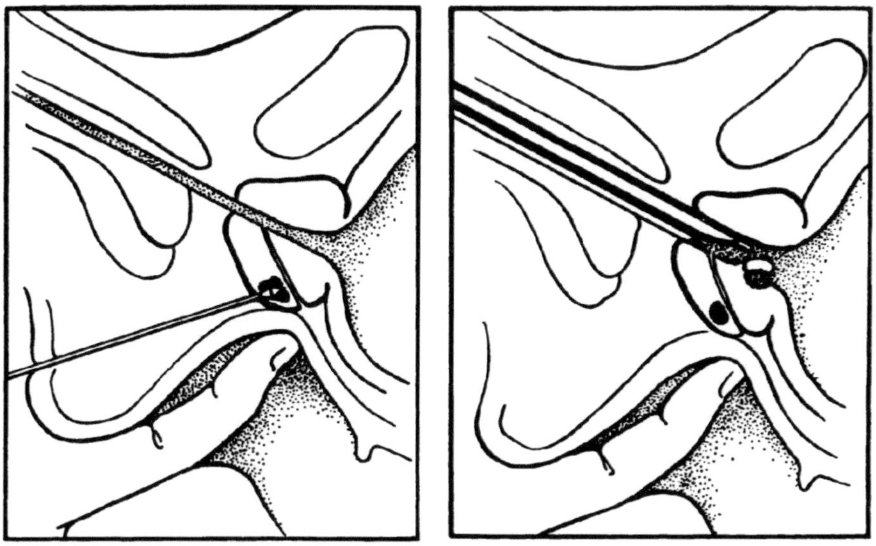

Fig. 7. The methods of perineal and transurethral prostate biopsies (Grabstald, 1965b)

5. Transrectal approach

By this period the usual procedure to obtain prostate biopsies was via the perineal route, however, the safety of transrectal approach was assured (Grabstald and Elliot, 1953; Grabstald, 1955 and 1956; Graham, 1958; Daves et al., 1961).

5.1 Transrectal needles: Aspiration and core biopsy

Various needles were used to collect tissue for cytological or histological diagnosis. Franzen et al. developed a fine needle and guide for prostatic aspiration by the transrectal route (figure 8). The Franzen needle and guide were designed to allow accurate needle placement into the abnormal area palpated by the fingertip. It was secured by the metal ring fixed to the fingertip and a plate in the palm of the hand. A rubber fingerstall was pulled over it and a 23- or 25-gauge needle was used. Up to six passes could be made in one session (Berner and Orell, 2010). Using this needle Williams et al. were able to achieve satisfactory results (Williams et al., 1967).

The Silverman needle, designed in 1938, was first to be used to take prostatic tissue by Peirson and Nickerson and they published their cohort of 36 patients (Peirson and Nickerson, 1943). They were able to achieve satisfactory histological specimens in 86% of cases.

A specific comparison of the Franzen and Silverman needles was undertaken by Hendry and Williams and their findings were published in 1971 (Hendry and Williams, 1971). The Franzen needle provided cytological diagnosis and carried advantages of causing less morbidity and could be carried out on an outpatient basis, however the likelihood of missing a cancer was greater compared with using the Silverman needle. The latter provided histological diagnosis and resulted in a lower false negative rate but required a general anaesthetic. Ultimately their recommendations were that the Franzen technique could be used as an initial investigation, however should the test prove negative then it could be repeated, and thereafter the urologist could proceed to the Silverman technique.

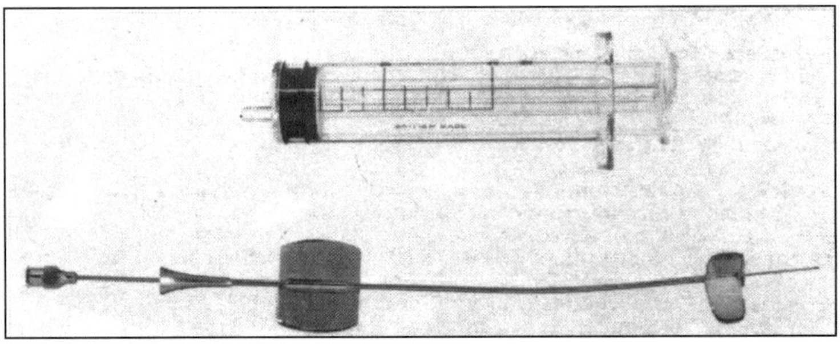

Fig. 8. The Franzen needle and guide with Gillette Scmitar disposable syringe

The Gillette Scmitar was found to be more effective at aspiration (Hendry and Williams, 1971) Other investigators found that using either the Franzen needle method or a larger bore needle to withdraw histological material produced equal chances of obtaining sufficient tissue for diagnosis (Andersson et al., 1967; Ekman et al., 1967). Furthermore Alfthan et al. documented that tissue obtained by needle aspiration was as reliable for diagnosis as histological samples produced by transperineal Silverman needle (Alfthan et al., 1968).

5.2 Digital-guidance

Finger-guided needle biopsy of the prostate through the rectum was used widely as a technique from the mid 1950s, although Astraldi can be credited with carrying out the first transrectal prostate biopsy (Astraldi, 1937). This approach offered more promise of diagnostic accuracy when sampling a prostatic nodule compared with perineal needle biopsy (Barnes, 1959).

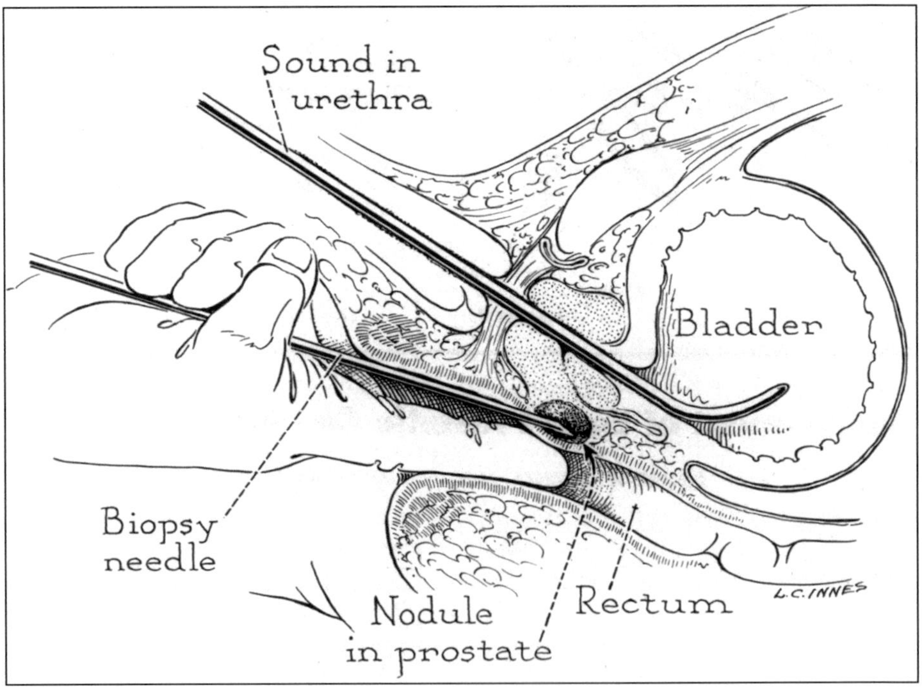

Fig. 9. Digitally-guided transrectal biopsy of the prostate with the aid of a urethral sound.

The sound in the urethra allowed the prostate to be directed posteriorly to facilitate palpation of the nodule and placement of the Silverman needle (Barnes & Emery, 1959).
The patient would be anaesthetized and positioned in lithotomy. An initial digital rectal examination (DRE) was performed to ensure an empty rectum and an ounce of antiseptic solution was instilled per rectally for ten minutes. Agents used included Vioform (iodochlorhydroxyquin U.S.P) 3% Betadine (providone-iodine) or Triophyll (tri-iodophynol). A sound was inserted transurethrally by an assistant to displace the prostate dorsally and towards the anal outlet (figure 10). With a gloved index finger inserted into the rectum with a Silverman biopsy needle applied close to the finger with the tip of the needle in line with the tip of the finger and the bevel edge facing away from the finger. The needle is then rotated half a turn so that the beveled edge is against the finger. This avoided an inadvertent needlestick injury. The abnormal area was palpated and the needle directed through the rectal mucosa and towards the area, but not into it. The obturator was then removed and a bivalved biopsy obturator was inserted through the needle and into the prostate. The bivalved biopsy obturator is held static whilst the needle is rotated and advanced about 1.5cm. The bivalved obturator is then removed from the needle and a core of tissue is taken from between its blades

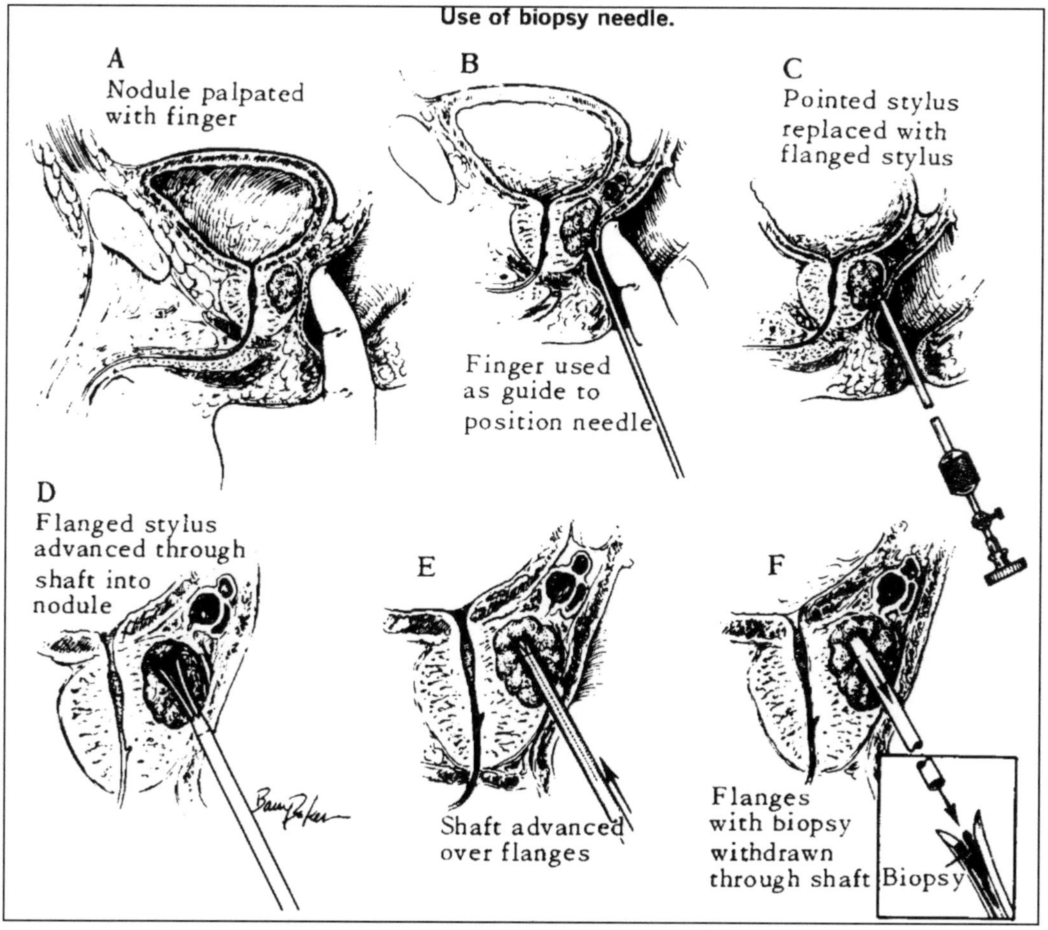

Fig. 10. Digital-guided transrectal biopsy of the prostate

5.3 Open transrectal biopsy

This method was performed using a proctotomy incision and the advantage of this was that it allowed access to the very portion of the prostate that was most often involved in cancer, the posterior lobe, and furthermore larger pieces of material could be extracted (figure 11) (Grabstald, 1965b). The drawback of the procedure was that subsequent radical surgery was difficult using the retropubic approach in terms of dissection and also cases of rectourethral fistulae had been reported (Grabstald, 1965b).

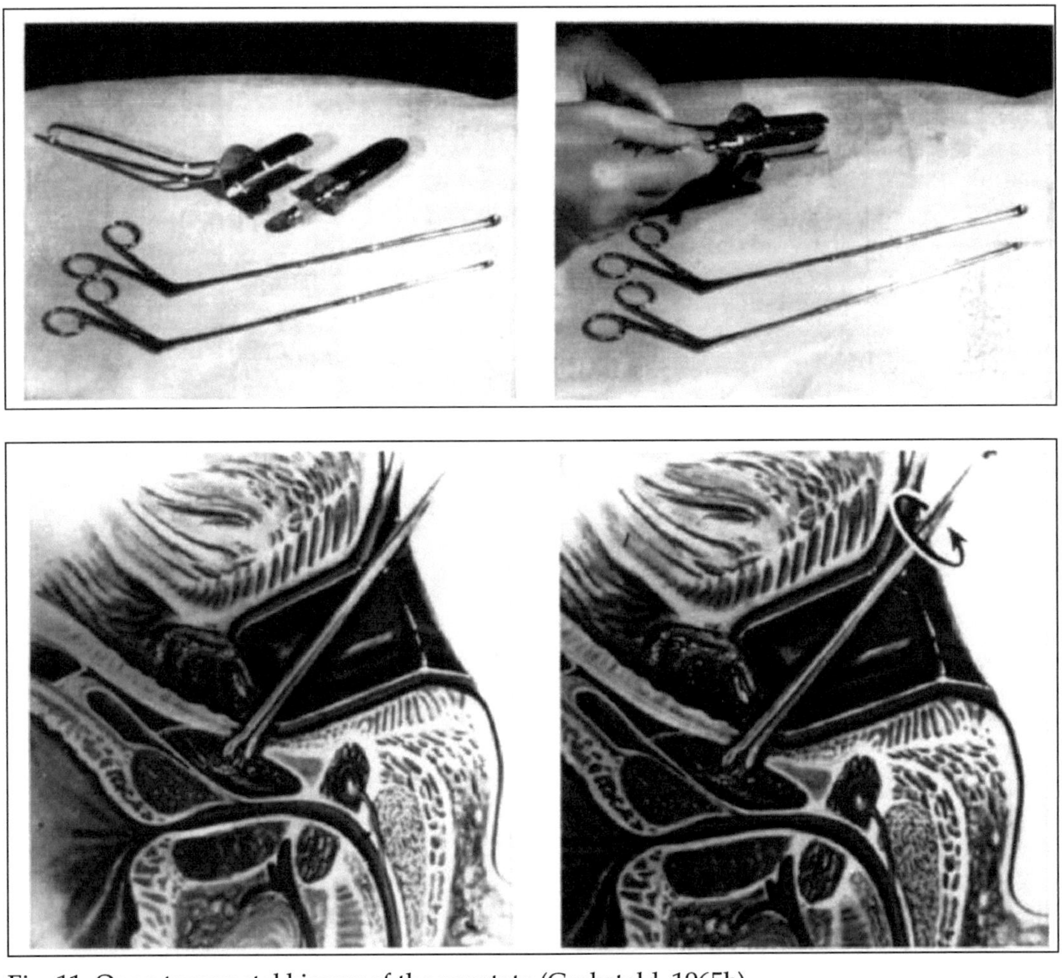

Fig. 11. Open transrectal biopsy of the prostate (Grabstald, 1965b)

5.4 Ultrasound-guided transrectal biopsy

5.4.1 The development of ultrasound imaging

Biopsy techniques continued to be digitally-guided until the development of ultrasound imaging. Takahashi and Ouchi were the first to describe the use of transrectal ultrasound to evaluate the prostate (Takahashi & Ouchi, 1963). However the image quality was too poor to be of any clinical use. It was Watanabe et al. who are credited with obtaining the first clinically useful transrectal images of the prostate. They used a 3.5MHz probe, which was considered to be state of the art at the time, although image quality was relatively poor (Watanabe et al., 1967).

It was not until the 1980s when technological advances in probe manufacture and the development of attachable biopsy apparatus that ultrasound became clinically useful for the diagnosis of prostate cancer. A 7MHz probe was developed allowing delineation of the architecture of the prostate and extensive research was carried out to identify sonographic appearances of prostate cancer. Concurrently serum prostate specific antigen (PSA) testing was introduced and elevated levels prompted further investigations.

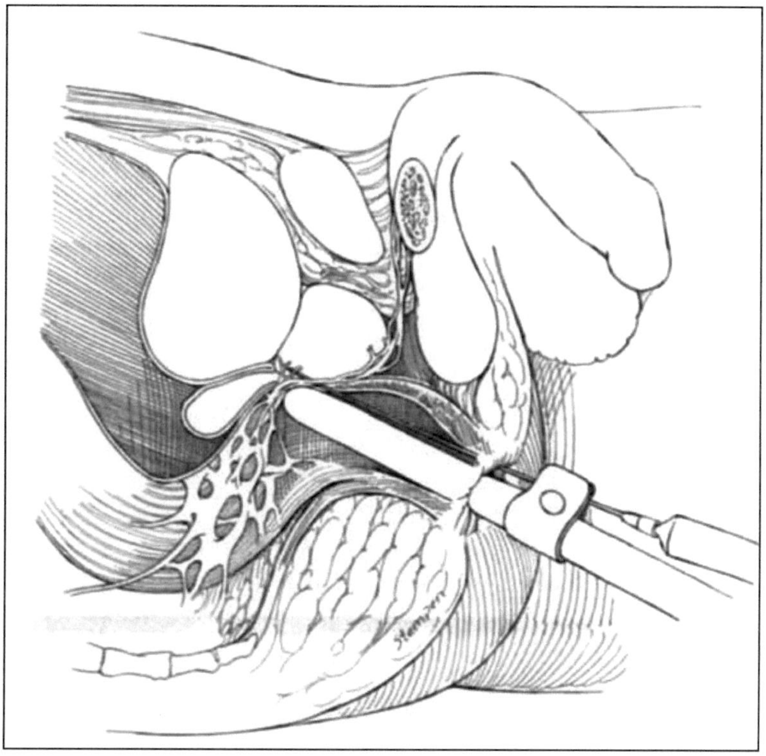

Fig. 12. Transrectal ultrasound probe in situ (Nash et al., 1996)

5.4.2 Sonographic appearances of prostate cancer

Detailed research on prostate anatomy was also carried out and McNeal proposed that the prostate was composed of three distinct glandular zones, namely transitional zone, peripheral zone and central zone (McNeal, 1968). The clinical relevance became important considering that the majority (70-80%) of cancers arise in the peripheral zone.

The findings of research into ultrasound appearances of prostate cancer confirmed varying characteristics and early stage lesions were seen to be indistinct from normal prostatic tissue, indicating that TRUS as a diagnostic tool lacked specificity and had limitations. With the widespread use of serum PSA testing came the detection of early stage, low volume cancers that did not necessarily have any palpable abnormality or specific sonographic findings. In response, the method of sampling the prostate gland had to change and that change occurred in 1989.

6. The modern era of prostate needle biopsy

6.1 The sextant method

In 1989, Hodge et al. published two papers in the *Journal of Urology* (Hodge et al., 1989a and 1989b). The first paper described directed transrectal prostate biopsies of palpable abnormalities, 90% of which had corresponding hypoechoic lesions on ultrasound (Hodge 1989a). Additional biopsies were also taken of isoechoic areas of the peripheral and central zones. These biopsies were not systematic and they were found to be positive in 66% of cases.

The second article was a landmark paper which marked the start of the modern era of prostate needle biopsy (Hodge et al., 1989b). Hodge et al. compared the use of transrectal prostate biopsies taken of palpable or sonographic abnormalities to those taken in a random systematic fashion. The latter method involved taking biopsies from six sites: the apex, middle and base of each prostate lobe, parasagitally, in addition to any hypoechoic lesion seen on ultrasound. This sextant technique detected 9% more cancers compared with the former method. As a result of this there was a shift away from lesion-directed biopsies to a method of systematic sampling of the prostate using transrectal ultrasound to guide accurate needle placement.

The Hodge protocol of systematic sextant biopsy of the prostate became the gold standard for many years in an era when an elevated PSA was an acceptable indication for prostate biopsy regardless of DRE findings.

6.2 Beyond sextant biopsies

Some years later Stamey modified the sextant technique and took sextant biopsies that were lateral to the mid-sagittal plane in the peripheral zone where most prostate cancers are typically located (Stamey, 1995). Other investigators went on to study alternatives to the traditional sextant biopsy, namely the optimum number of core biopsies for diagnosis as well as sampling of the transition zone in an effort to improve the negative predictive value of prostate biopsy.

Intuitively researchers began sampling more prostatic tissue however the procedure was not without pain. Sixty-five to 90% of patients experienced discomfort (Clements et al., 1993; Collins et al., 1993) and this discomfort was proportional to number of cores taken (Nash et al., 1996). A pioneering report published by Nash et al. provided evidence that effective pain relief could be achieved by infiltrating local anaesthetic (Nash et al., 1996). And so with the introduction of the peri-prostatic nerve blockade it became possible to take 10 to 18 or even 20 biopsies.

Eskew et al. introduced the systematic extended biopsy technique and described the 5-region biopsy protocol whereby conventional sextant biopsies were taken along with two additional cores from the far lateral portion of each side and three centralized cores (Eskew et al., 1997). When the prostate gland was over 50cc, one additional core is taken per region. Thirty-five percent of those patients diagnosed with prostate cancer were found to have cancers in the extra five biopsies sites and not in the sextant regions. Eighty-eight percent of those were located in the far lateral zones, 12% in the central zone.

Levine et al. published a series which involved 137 men with abnormal DRE findings or a raised serum PSA. These patients underwent two independent consecutive sets of sextant biopsies at the same sitting (Levine et al., 1999). They showed an increase in prostate cancer detection from 21% in sextant biopsy alone to 31% with the additional six biopsies.

Presti et al. took two extra biopsies laterally on each side at the base and mid gland in addition to the traditional sextant technique in an effort to include more peripheral zone tissue in their sampling (Presti et al., 2000). This produced a 10-core biopsy. They enrolled 483 men with either abnormal DRE or a PSA ≥4 ng/mL. On analysis of the cancer detection rate from each side, it was discovered that the traditional sextant technique missed 20% of cancers. Eight cancers were missed by the 10-biopsy scheme and were detected by lesion-directed or transition zone biopsies instead, for a detection rate of 96%. By eliminating the sextant base biopsies, the detection rate was 95%. Therefore the authors concluded that the optimum protocol was an 8-core biopsy scheme.

An 11-core biopsy protocol was investigated by Babaian et al. and involved using the traditional sextant sites as well as the anterior horn on each side (lateral anterior peripheral zone), transition zone on each side (anterior to and next to the urethra), and one mid-gland biopsy (Babaian et al., 2000). A 33% increase in prostate cancer was found using these additional zones, with the anterior horn being the most frequently positive biopsy site.

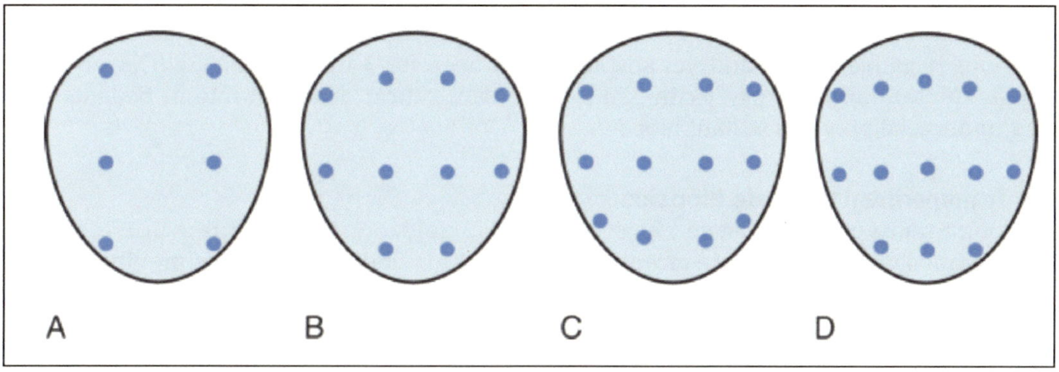

Fig. 13. Various reported systematic biopsy schemes.
Base is at the top of the figure, apex is at the bottom.
A. Sextant biopsy scheme originally proposed by Hodge et al.; B. The 10-core biopsy of Presti et al.; C. The 12-core, or double sextant biopsy of Levine et al. D. The 13-core, 5-region biopsy of Eskew et al. (Wein et al., 2007)

Studies were also carried out on digitally-reconstructed radical prostatectomy specimens which showed the inadequacy of the traditional sextant biopsy method. In one study by Chen et al., simulation biopsy strategies were conducted on whole-mount radical prostatectomy specimens from 180 patients and it was found that only 73% of cancers were detected by sextant biopsy (Chen et al., 1997). Using a 10-core biopsy scheme, incorporating the midline peripheral zone, the inferior portion of the anterior horn of the peripheral zone, and the transition zone, they picked up 96% of cancers with a volume ≥0.5cc (clinically significant).

Bauer et al. studied 201 step-sectioned whole mount radical prostatectomy specimens and mapped out the location of the cancers using a 3-dimensional computer simulation (Bauer et al., 1999). They calculated that a 10- or 12-core, laterally-directed biopsy protocol would detect 99% of the cancers, while the traditional sextant protocol would detect only 72.6%.

One of the concerns of increasing the number of prostate biopsies was causing the patient increased discomfort. Naughton et al. carried out a prospective randomized study to assess the pain and morbidity associated with 6 biopsies compared with 12 (Naughton et al., 2000). They concluded that there was no difference in the discomfort experienced, and no increase rate in moderate or major problems, although there was a higher rate of haematospermia (89% versus 71%) and rectal bleeding (24% versus 10%).

6.3 Saturation biopsies

With increasing number of cores came the concept of saturation biopsy, a term coined by Stewart et al. (Stewart et al., 2001), in which 20 or more systematic cores were taken. Djavan et al. developed tables to recommend more cores for larger glands, but these met with little clinical acceptance (Djavan et al., 1999).

These saturation biopsies have been offered to those who have had previous negative biopsies but continue to have clinical suspicion for prostate cancer. This technique is generally not considered as an initial biopsy strategy since the cancer detection rates compared with extended protocols is no greater (de la Taille et al., 2003; Guichard et al., 2007).

In a series by Djavan et al. a 24-core biopsy template was used in 116 patients with a previous negative biopsy and yet suspicious findings for a missed tumour (Djavan et al., 2001). The saturation biopsy technique noted a 41% cancer detection rate in patients who had undergone previous sextant biopsy.

6.4 Transperineal template biopsies

Although transperineal prostate biopsy with TRUS guidance was described in 1981 (Holm and Gammelgaard, 1981), more recent research has been undertaken on this previously used transperineal approach with the additional use of templates. This has facilitated control of the biopsy gun and allowed uniform sampling of the whole prostate. Furthermore there has been growing interest in the use of brachytherapy grid to take transperineal biopsies and therefore saturate the entire gland. Fewer complications have been reported with this technique and yet a greater detection rate of prostate cancer.

7. Conclusion

The history of the development of prostate biopsy has changed significantly from random biopsies, to systematic to extended biopsy schemes. Systematic sextant biopsies, even when laterally directed, do not provide adequate sampling of the prostate. Ultimately the sextant biopsy technique has now become obsolete in favour of more extended biopsy protocols. To date there is no consensus on the optimal number of cores without significantly increasing morbidity but it has been shown that as prostate gland size increases, the yield of sextant biopsy has decreased (Karakiewicz et al., 1997). Based on published data it appears that between 8 and 12 cores would be an acceptable protocol.

Essentially the role of TRUS as an imaging tool of the prostate remains vital for accurate needle placement and sampling of the prostate as well as taking volume measurement. TRUS technology has also become the mainstay of other image-guided prostate interventions such as brachytherapy, cryotherapy and high-intensity frequency ultrasound (HIFU), as well as being used in the evaluation of appropriate patients for treatment of benign prostatic hyperplasia (Beerlage, 2003).

8. References

Aarnink, R.G., Beerlage, H.P., de la Rosette, J.J. et al. Transrectal ultrasound of the prostate: innovations and future applications. J Urol. 1998; 159: 1568-1579

Alfthan, O., Klintrup, H.E., Koivuniemi, A. et al. Comparison of thin-needle and Vim-Silverman-needle biopsy in the diagnosis of prostatic cancer. Duodecim. 1968; 84: 506

Andersson, L., Jonsson, G. and Brunk, U. Puncture biopsy of the prostate in the diagnosis of prostatic cancer. Scand J Urol and Neph. 1967; 1: 227

Applewhite, J.C., Matlaga, B.R, McCullough, D.L. et al. Transrectal ultrasound and biopsy in early diagnosis of prostate cancer. Cancer Control. 2001; 8(2): 141-150

Astraldi, A. Diagnosis of cancer of the prostate: biopsy by rectal route. Urol Cutan Rev. 1937; 41: 421–427

Babaian, RJ, Toi, A., Kamoi, K., et al. A comparative analysis of sextant and an extended 11-core multisite directed biopsy Strategy. J Urol. 2000; 163: 152–157

Barnes, R.W. and Emery, D.S. Management of early prostatic carcinoma. Calif Med. 1959; 91(2): 57-61

Barringer, B.S. Carcinoma of the prostate. Surg Gynecol Obstet. 1922; 34: 168–176

Barringer, B.S. Prostatic carcinoma. J Urol. 1942; 47: 306–310

Bauer, J.J., Zeng, J., Weir, J., et al. Three-dimensional computer-simulated prostate models: Lateral prostate biopsies increase the detection rate of prostate cancer. Urology. 1999; 53: 961–967

Beerlage, H.P. Alternative therapies for localized prostate cancer. Curr Urol Rep 2003; 4: 216-220

Berner, A. and Orell, S.R. Prostate gland, In: Diagnostic Cytopathology, Gray W and Kocjan G (Ed.), 527-536. ISBN 0702031542, 9780702031540, Elsevier Health Sciences, Churchill Livingstone, 2010

Boyd, M.L., Nuckolls, J.B. Carcinoma of the prostate. J Med Assoc Georgia. 1940; 29: 493–499

Chen, M.E., Troncoso, P., Johnston, D.A., et al. Optimization of prostate biopsy strategy using computer based analysis. J Urol. 1997; 158: 2168–2175

Clements, R., Aideyan, O.U., Griffiths, G.J. et al. Side effects and patient acceptability of transrectal biopsy of the prostate. Clin. Rad. 1993; 47: 125

Colby, F.H. Carcinoma of the prostate: results of the total prostatectomy. J Urol. 1953; 69: 797–806

Collins, G.N, Lloyd, S.N., Hehir, M. et al. Multiple transrectal ultrasound-guided prostatic biopsies - true morbidity and patient acceptance. BJU. 1993; 71: 460

Daves, J.A., Tomskey, G.C., and Cohen, A.E. Transrectal needle biopsy of the prostate. J Urol. 1961; 85: 180

de la Taille, A., Antiphon, P., Salomon, L., et al. Prospective evaluation of a 21-sample needle biopsy procedure designed to improve the prostate cancer detection rate. Urology 2003; 61: 1181–1186

Denton, S.E., Valk, W.L., Jacobson, J.M. et al. Comparison of the perineal needle biopsy and the transurethral prostatectomy in the diagnosis of prostatic carcinoma: an analysis of 300 cases. J Urol. 1967; 97: 127

Djavan, B., Zlotta, A.R., Remzi, M., et al. Total and transition zone prostate volume and age: how do they affect the utility of PSA-based diagnostic parameters for early prostate cancer detection? Urology 1999; 54: 846–852

Djavan. B., Ravery, V. and Ziotta, A.R. Prospective evaluation of prostate cancer detected on biopsies 1, 2, 3 and 4: when should we stop? J Urol. 2001; 166: 1269–1283

Ekman, H., Hedberg, K. and Person, P.S. Cytological versus histological examination of needle biopsy specimens in the diagnosis of prostatic cancer. BJU. 1967; 39: 544

Eskew, L.A., Bare, R.L. and McCullough, D.L. Systematic 5 region prostate biopsy is superior to sextant method for diagnosing carcinoma of the prostate. J Urol. 1997; 157: 199–202

Ferguson, R.S. Prostatic neoplasms: their diagnosis by needle puncture and aspiration. Am J Surg 1930; 9: 507–511

Ferguson, R.S. Diagnosis and treatment of early carcinoma of the prostate. J Urol. 1937; 37: 774–782

Grabstald, H. Further experience with transrectal biopsy of the prostate. J Urol. 1955; 74: 211-212

Grabstald, H. Summary of currently employed prostatic biopsy methods, with comments concerning combined transrectal biopsy and radical retropubic prostatectomy. BJU. 1956; 28: 176.

Grabstald, H. The clinical and laboratory diagnosis of cancer of the prostate. A Cancer Journal for Clinicians; 1965a: 15: 76-81

Grabstald, H. Biopsy techniques in the diagnosis of cancer of the prostate. A Cancer Journal for Clinicians; 1965b: 15: 134–138

Grabstald, H. The incidence, clinical and pathological classification of cancer of the prostate. A Cancer Journal for Clinicians. 1965c; 15: 31–35

Grabstald, H. and Elliott, J.L. Transrectal biopsy of the prostate. JAMA. 1953; 153, 563

Graham, W.H. Carcinoma of the prostate. BJU. 1958; 30: 389

Guichard, G., Larre, S., Gallina, A., et al. Extended 21-sample needle biopsy protocol for diagnosis of prostate cancer in 1000 consecutive patients. Eur Urol 2007; 52: 430–435

Heidenreich, A., Bolla, M., Joniau, S. et al. Guidelines on prostate cancer. European Association of Urology, 2010

Hendry, W.F. and Williams, J.P. Transrectal Prostatic Biopsy. BMJ. 1971; 4: 595-597

Hodge, K.K., McNeal, J.E., Stamey, T.A. Ultrasound guided transrectal core biopsies of the palpably abnormal prostate. J Urol. 1989a; 142: 66–7

Hodge, K.K., McNeal, J.E., Terris, M.K., et al. Random systematic versus directed ultrasound guided transrectal core biopsies of the prostate. J Urol. 1989b; 142: 71–74

Holm, H.H. and Gammelgaard, J. Ultrasonically guided precise needle placement in the prostate and the seminal vesicles. J Urol. 1981; 126: 385

Huggins, C., and Johnson, M.A.. Cancer of the bladder and prostate. JAMA. 1947; 135: 1146-1152

Jewett, H.J. The present status of radical prostatectomy for stages A and B prostatic cancer. Urol Clin N Am. 1975; 2: 105

Karakiewicz, P.I., Bazinet, M., Aprikian, A.G., et al. Outcome of sextant biopsy according to gland volume. Urology 1997; 49:55–59

Kaufman, J.J., Rosenthal, M. and Goodwin, W.E.. Needle biopsy in diagnosis of prostate cancer. California Medicine. 1954; 81; 5: 308-313

Levine, M.A., Ittman, M., Melamed, J., et al. Two consecutive sets of transrectal ultrasound guided sextant biopsies of the prostate for thedetection of prostate cancer. J Urol. 1998; 159: 471–475

McNeal, J.E. Regional morphology and pathology of the prostate. Am J Clin Pathol. 1968; 49: 347

Nash, P.A., Bruce, J.E., Indudhara, R. et al. Transrectal ultrasound guided prostatic nerve blockade eases systematic needle biopsy of the prostate. J Urol. 1996; 155: 607-609

Naughton, C.K., Ornstein, D.K., Smith, D.S., et al. Pain and morbidity of transrectal ultrasound guided prostate biopsy: A prospective randomized trial of 6 versus 12 cores. J Urol. 2000; 163: 168–171

Parry, W.L., and Finelli, J.F. Biopsy of the prostate. J Urol. 1960; 84: 643–648

Peirson, E.L. and Nickerson, D.A.: Biopsy of the prostate with the Silverman Needle. N Engl J Med. 1943; 228: 675-678

Presti, J.C., Chang, J.J., Bhargava, V., et al: The optimal systematic prostate biopsy scheme should include 8 rather than 6 biopsies: results of a prospective clinical trial. J Urol. 2000; 163: 163–166

Purser, B.N., Robinson, B.C., and Mostofi, F.K. Comparison of needle biopsy and transurethral resection biopsy in the diagnosis of carcinoma of the prostate. J Urol. 1967; 98, 224

Scattoni, V., Maccagnano, C., Zanni, G. et al. Is extended and saturation biopsy necessary? Int J Urol. 2010; 17: 432–47

Silletti, J.P., Gordon, G.J., Bueno, R. et al. Prostate biopsy: Past, present and future. Urology. 2007; 69: 413-416

Smith, J.A. Jr. Transrectal ultrasonography for the detection and staging of carcinoma of the prostate. J Clin Ultrasound. 1996; 24: 455-461

Stamey, T.A. Making the most out of six systematic sextant biopsies. Urology 1995; 45: 2–12

Stewart, C.S., Leibovich, B.C., Weaver, A.L. et al. Prostate cancer diagnosis using a saturation needle biopsy technique after previous negative sextant biopsies. J Urol. 2001; 166: 1, 86–91

Takahashi, H. and Ouchi, T. The ultrasonic diagnosis in the field of urology. Proc Jpn Soc Ultrasonics Med. 1963; 3: 7

Watanabe, H., Igari, D., Tanahasi, Y., et al. Development and application of new equipment for transrectal ultrasonography. J Clin Ultrasound. 1974; 2: 91-98

Wein, A.J., Kavoussi, L.R., Novick, A.C., et al (Ed.). Campbell-Walsh Urology. Saunders Elsevier. ISBN 13: 978-0-8089-2353-4. 9th Ed, 2007

Whitmore, W.F., Jr. Hormone therapy in prostate cancer. Am J Med. 1956; 21: 697

Wild, J.J., Reid, J.M. Progress in techniques of soft tissue examination by 15 MC pulsed ultrasound. In: Kelley-Fry E, ed. Ultrasound in biology and medicine: a symposium sponsored by the Bioacoustics Laboratory of the University of Illinois and the Physiology Branch of the Office of Naval Research. Robert Allerton Park, Monticello, Ill; June 20-22, 1955. Washington, DC: American Institute of Biological Sciences; 1957: 30-45

Williams, J.P., Still, B.M., and Pugh, R.C.B. The diagnosis of prostatic cancer: cytological and biochemical studies using the franzen biopsy needle. BJU. 1967; 39: 549

Young, H.H. and Davis, D.M.: Young's Practice of Urology. Philadelphia, WB Saunders, 1926; 2: 414–512

2

Radical Transurethral Resection of the Prostate: A Possible Radical Procedure Against Localized Prostate Cancer with Almost No Postoperative Urinary Incontinence

Masaru Morita and Takeshi Matsuura
Kounaizaka Clinic, Matsubara Tokushukai Hospital
Japan

1. Introduction

Current radical surgery against localized prostate cancer (PCa), such as open (Memmelaar, 1949; Reiner & Walsh, 1979; Walsh & Donker, 1982), laparoscopic (Schuessler et al., 1997; Abbou et al., 2000; Guillonneau et al., 2003) or robot-assisted prostatectomy (Binder & Kramer, 2001; Menon et al., 2002; Menon et al., 2004), has a possible risk to injure supporting structures that surround and support the prostate as well as the external sphincter and the neurovascular bundle. As a result, postoperative stress urinary incontinence develops and continues in about 10 % of patients (Stanford et al., 2000; Lepor et al., 2004; Namiki et al., 2009; Menon et al., 2007). Many procedures were introduced to improve the recovery of postoperative sexual function and urinary incontinence: bladder neck suspension or reconstruction (Poon et al., 2000), reconstruction of the rhabdosphincter (Rocco et al., 2007), periurethral suspension of the dorsal vein complex/urethral complex (Patel et al., 2009) and preservation of the neurovascular bundle (Kaiho et al., 2005), but have failed to solve the problems completely until now.

The idea of a transurethral approach to resect almost total prostate tissues containing prostate cancer dates back to around 1990 (Valdivia Uría & López López, 1989; Reuter et al., 1991). The technique did not significantly increase the operative morbidity and mortality compared with transurethral resection of the prostate (TURP) for benign prostate hyperplasia (BPH), and was suggested to be a valid alternative in some patients with prostate cancer. And a recent report concluded that localized prostate cancer could be resected transurethrally as radical as open surgery (Reuter et al., 2008).

We thought that the transurethral approach to treat prostate cancer might bring better clinical results in the era of more improved resectoscope and more sensitive PSA test for the follow-up examination. We applied the transurethral technique to manage prostate cancer with the intention to eliminate almost all prostate tissues that contained localized cancer. As we already reported (Morita & Matsuura, 2009), radical transurethral resection of prostate cancer (RTUR-PCa) against localized prostate cancer has a possibility to minimize the injury to the external sphincter because an operator is able to recognize it clearly during the operation. With a minimal injury to the supporting structures of the prostate, we think that urinary continence can be reserved in RTUR-PCa at least at a similar rate in transurethral resection of the prostate for BPH. Urinary incontinence after TURP is reported to occur in 0.4 – 3.3 % of the patients (Holtgrewe et al., 1989; AUA Practice Guidelines Committee, 2003).

2. Patients and methods

2.1 Patients

Between December 2003 and December 2007, a total of 222 radical transurethral resection of prostate cancer were performed under spinal anesthesia in 170 patients with clinical stages of T1 or T2. Clinical stages were determined according to the UICC TNM staging system of 1997. We informed the patients that the procedure was not a current standard radical method of management, and those who refused this procedure were excluded from the study. We also excluded patients with serious comorbidities that might affect their lives by standard TURP. Patients who gave a written informed consent were eligible for the study in the order they were given a diagnosis of localized prostate cancer. Institutional review board approved the TUR-PCa program after the preliminary study.

Clinical stage was determined mainly by digital rectal examination and transrectal ultrasonography combined with the result of needle biopsy. We selected the patients to be checked for metastasis by eliminating patients with a minimum risk of metastasis according to Partin nomogram (Partin et al., 1993) and other reports on bone metastasis (Oesterling, 1991; Oesterling, 1993). Ultrasound guided transrectal needle biopsy was performed on 123 patients under caudal block, excluding the patients who were given a diagnosis of PCa after transurethral resection of the prostate for BPH. We obtained a total of 14 samples per case from the peripheral and transition zone including far lateral part, dividing the prostate into base (2 cores), upper middle part (2 cores), lower middle part (6 cores) and apex (4 cores), and we marked at the dorsal end.

Patients ranged from 52 to 91 years old (mean ± SD: 72.9 ± 7.3, median: 74.0), preoperative PSA 1.5 to 100.5 ng/mL (mean ± SD: 10.38 ± 11.95, median: 6.2). Out of 170 patients, 20 patients were lost to follow-up, leaving 150 patient included in this study. Clinical stages were as follows: T1b: 39 cases, T1c: 88 cases, T2: 23 cases. The present study includes the patients who were given a diagnosis of prostate cancer after TURP for BPH and on antiandrogen therapy. Thirty-five patients with a clinical stage of T1b were on oral antiandrogen (chlormadinone acetate) therapy for a mean period of 72.1 weeks with the longest case for 12 years preoperatively. In 11 patients with a clinical stage of T1c, oral antiandrogen was administered for the period between 5 and 47 months (mean 23.0 months). In the other patients, oral antiandrogen was administered for 1 to 2 weeks just before RTUR-PCa, with no hormonal therapy being done after the operation.

2.2 Operative procedures

One authorized urologist (M.M.) performed all the operations. We used a standard TURP setup with an irrigation pressure of 80 cmH_2O and an irrigation rate of 250 ml/min using D-sorbitol solution. After a rough resection of almost all the transition and central zone, we tried to resect and fulgurate the peripheral zone as completely as possible, especially where cancer was detected by biopsy. The resection was continued until adipose tissue, venous sinus or the external sphincter was identified. But we did not resect prostate tissues until adipose tissue was exposed all around the operative field. We aggressively fulgurated the area adjacent to where adipose tissue was exposed because the remaining prostate tissue could be considered a thin layer. We especially paid attention not to distend the bladder too much to prevent a high irrigation pressure and a resultant TUR syndrome. Special attention was paid to avoid the injury to Santorini's plexus and the rectum. The procedure was started from the 12 o'clock position, dividing the prostate into 6 parts, and resected specimens were collected separately to examine the distribution of cancer. The seminal vesicle was partially resected at its attached part to the prostate between the 4 and 8 o'clock positions to determine the invasion of cancer. Finally the verumontanum was resected to achieve the complete resection of prostate tissue. A bag catheter was removed on the third postoperative day.

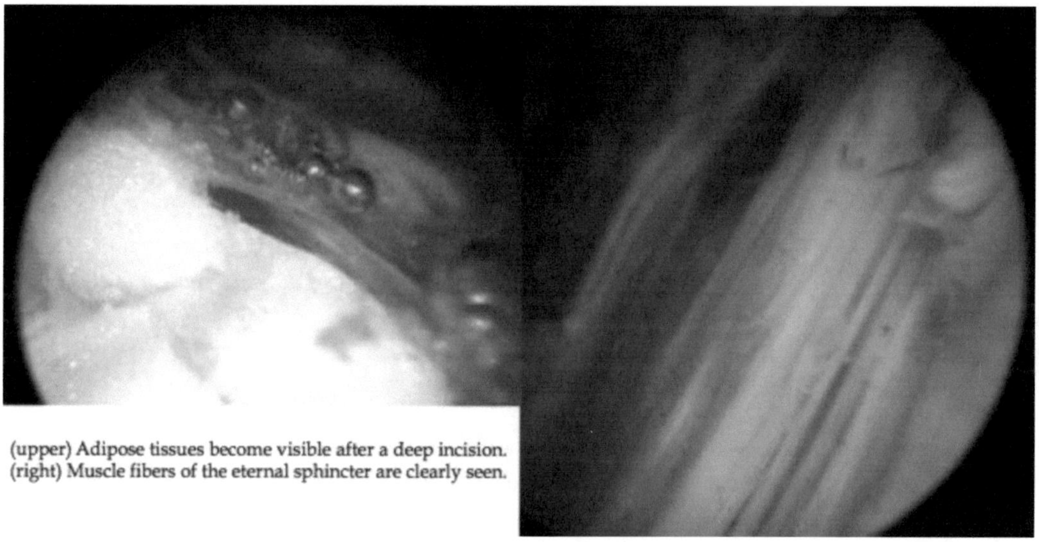

Fig. 1. As radical TUR proceeds, adipose tissue and the external sphincter can be seen.

2.3 Follow-up

Postoperative PSA was measured every two months starting two months after the initial operation. PSA failure was diagnosed when PSA showed a consecutive rise over 0.2 ng/mL. This was also applied to the indication of the second RTUR-PCa. But when the PSA level reached a plateau between 0.2 and 1.0 ng/mL, we did not think immediately that the patients were in a treatment failure.

3. Results

3.1 Results of RTUR-PCa

The mean follow up period of 150 patients was 45.1 ± 13.1 months (median: 43.9, range: 11 - 72 months). The operation time ranged between 60 and 125 min. (mean 80 min.), and the resected tissue weight was between 4.0 and 63.0 grams (mean ± SD: 15.1 ± 8.5, median: 14.0). The preoperative mean PSA value was 9.4 ± 9.7 ng/mL (median: 6.0, range: 1.5 to 66.3), with an unknown value in one patient. Pathological stages were as follows: pT2a: 60 cases, pT2b: 84, pT3: 5, pT4: 1 (Table 1). And Gleason score were: 4: 3 cases, 5: 7, 6: 35, 7: 67, 8: 17, 9: 21

(Table 2). Out of 20 patients who were lost to follow up, eight patients went for treatments elsewhere, five patients refused the second RTUR-PCa, and seven patients did not return to the clinic after their discharge. Three out of 8 patients who went to other hospitals underwent open radical prostatectomy. No malignant cells were detected pathologically in the residual prostate tissue in one patient, and no prostate tissue was found in the other two patients. Seven patients died during the follow-up period: three died of pneumonia, another of heart disease, of cerebrovascular accident, and of gastric cancer, and the last of biliary duct cancer, but there was no prostate cancer-related death. At present, ninety-seven patients have stable PSA after the first RTUR-PCa.

Pathological Stage	Total Patients		Patients treated with 1 operation				Patients treated with 2 operations			
	No. Patient	Preop PSA Mean(SD) Median(Range)	No. Patient	Patients with stable PSA after TUR: No. Patient	Patients with stable PSA after TUR: Latest PSA Mean(SD) Median(Range)	No. PSA Failure	No. Patient	Patients with stable PSA after TUR: No. Patient	Patients with stable PSA after TUR: Latest PSA Mean(SD) Median(Range)	No. PSA Failure
pT2a	60	7.84(9.13) 4.90(1.50-66.30)	45	43	0.080(0.138) 0.019(0.001-0.685)	2	15	12	0.018(0.025) 0.008(0.001-0.084)	3
pT2b	84	9.84 (9.69) 6.10(1.55-55.50)	53	53	0.071(0.108) 0.019(0.001-0.521)	2	29	24	0.052(0.090) 0.016(0.001-0.390)	5
pT3	5	11.60(5.90) 7.41(7.30-19.52)	3	1	0.001	2	2	1	0.484	1
pT4	1	43.80	1	0	-	1	0	0	-	0

Table 1. Results of RTUR-PCa grouped by pathological stage

Gleason Score	Total Patients		Patients treated with 1 operation				Patients treated with 2 operations			
	No. Patient	Preop PSA Mean(SD) Median(Range)	No. Patient	Patients with stable PSA after TUR: No. Patient	Patients with stable PSA after TUR: Latest PSA Mean(SD) Median(Range)	No. PSA Failure	No. Patient	Patients with stable PSA after TUR: No. Patient	Patients with stable PSA after TUR: Latest PSA Mean(SD) Median(Range)	No. PSA Failure
4	3	4.59(1.04) 4.41(3.65-5.70)	3	3	0.046(0.055) 0.016(0.012-0.11)	0	0	0	-	0
5	7	4.86(2.66) 4.40(1.90-8.90)	4	4	0.048(0.078) 0.013(0.002-0.165)	0	3	3	0.005(0.007) 0.016(0.001-0.013)	0
6	35	5.84(3.64) 4.69(1.50-21.4)	26	26	0.104(0.165) 0.032(0.001-0.685)	0	9	9	0.023(0.035) 0.005(0.001-0.094)	0
7	67	9.04(8.18) 6.00(3.14-55.50)	43	42	0.053(0.086) 0.013(0.001-0.305)	1	24	17	0.033(0.057) 0.008(0.001-0.241)	7
8	17	11.96(15.84) 7.30(2.59-66.30)	15	13	0.09640.090) 0.016(0.001-0.268)	2	2	2	0.205(0.262) 0.205(0.0019-0.390)	0
9	21	16.02(13.16) 11.60(3.50-44.10)	13	9	0.122(0.172) 0.045(0.001-0.521)	4	8	6	0.129(0.178) 0.069(0.001-0.484)	2

Table 2. Results of RTUR-PCa grouped by Gleason's score

The second TUR-PCa was performed in 46 patients between 5 and 51 months (mean 16.8) after the first operation. The resected tissue weight was between 5.0 and 14.0 grams (mean ± SD: 6.6 ± 1.3, median: 6.0). No cancer cells were detected pathologically in 13 patients (28.3 %). PSA failure was diagnosed in 9 patients who underwent the second RTUR-PCa. These patients showed high preoperative mean PSA value of 22.4 ng/mL (7.7 to 55.5 ng/mL) and PSA values did not fall significantly after the second RTUR-PCa. In the other 36 patents PSA levels stabilized after the second operation showing PSA≦0.01: 19 cases, ≦0.02: 4, ≦0.03: 2, ≦0.1: 7, ≦0.2: 1, ≦0.3: 1, ≦0.5: 2.

3.2 Overall results

PSA failure finally developed in 16 patients (10.7%) in the most recent follow-up. Preoperative PSA levels in these patients ranged from 7.3 to 55.5 ng/mL (mean 21.9), and Gleason scores were 7 in 8 patients, 8 in 2, and 9 in 6 (Table 1, 2). In the other 134 patients, PSA values stabilized as follows: PSA≦0.01: 55 cases, ≦0.02: 18, ≦0.03: 10, ≦0.04: 3, ≦0.1: 22, ≦0.2: 10, ≦0.7: 16.

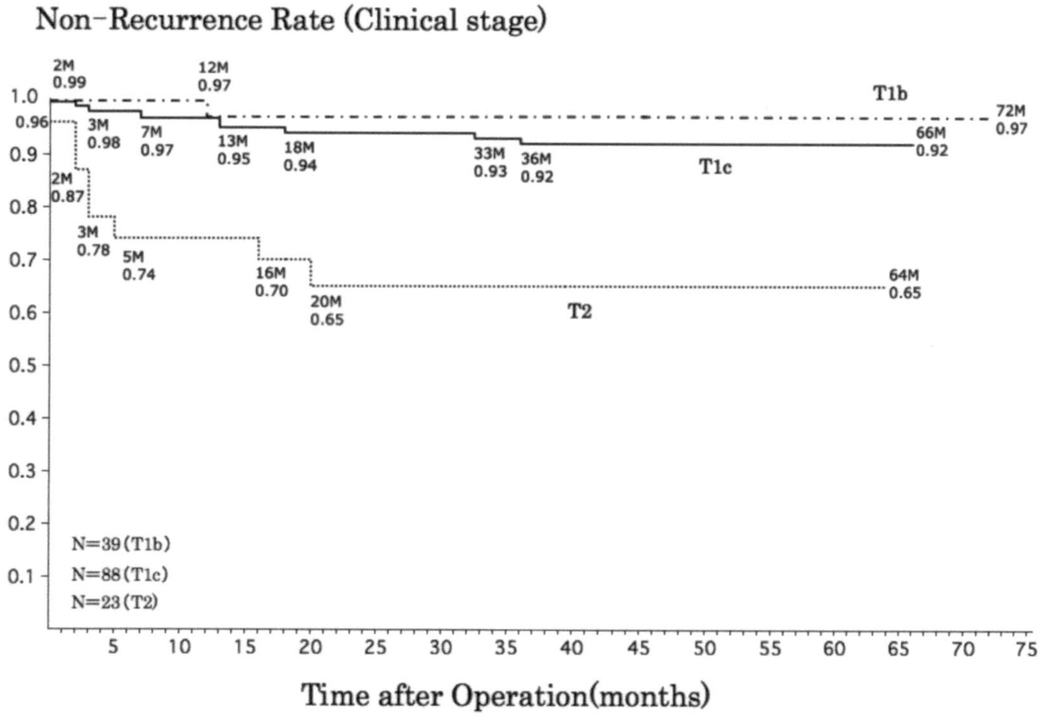

Fig. 2. Actuarial biochemical non-recurrence rate of each clinical stage

In all cases studied, the actuarial biological non-recurrence rate for each clinical stage were as follows: T1b: 0.97 at 72 months, T1c: 0.92 at 66 months, T2: 0.65 at 64 months (Fig. 2). The actuarial biological non-recurrence rate for pT2a at 66 months and pT2b at 72 months were 0.92 in both groups (Fig. 3).

Non-recurrence rate of each risk group according to D'Amico classification (D'Amico et.al, 1998) are shown in Fig. 4. PSA failure did not develop in the low-risk group of 34 patients (stage T1c, T2a and PSA level≦10 ng/mL and Gleason score≦6). Biological non-recurrence rate was 91.4 % in the intermediate-risk group of 70 patients (stage T2b or Gleason score of 7 or 10<PSA level≦20 ng/mL) and 78.3 % in the high-risk group of 46 patients (stage T2c or PSA level>20 ng/mL or Gleason score≧8) respectively.

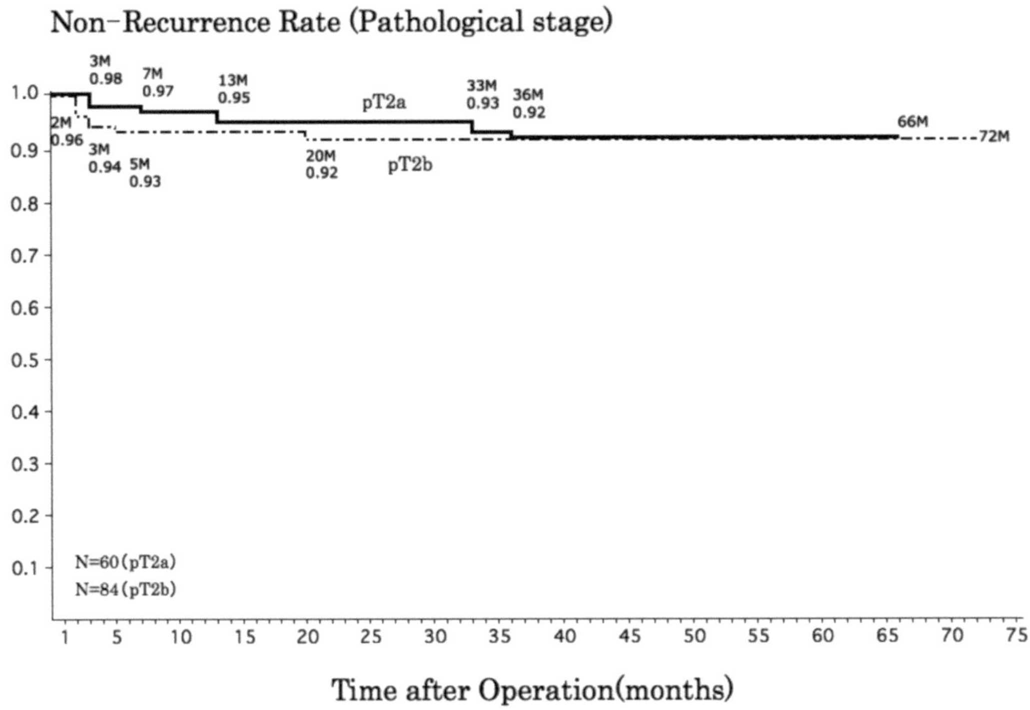

Fig. 3. Actuarial biochemical non-recurrence rate of each pathological stage (pT2a, solid line; pT2b, dotted line)

3.3 Learning curve

In some of the patients that underwent the first operation until March 2006, the PSA level did not show a sufficient drop. The operative technique became proficient and stable after that time, resulting in an acceptable clinical outcome (Fig. 5). Only 8 cases needed the second operation in 73 cases ($p<0.0001$ compared with cases before March 2006, chi square test) including 7 cases of PSA failure and 2 cases that was lost to follow-up, yielding more cases with lower PSA level as follows: PSA≤0.01: 31 cases, ≤0.02: 15, ≤0.03: 4, ≤0.04: 2, ≤0.1: 8, ≤0.2: 4, ≤0.6: 3. Nadir PSA levels were 0.013 ± 0.026 ng/mL (median, 0.004; range, 0.001-0.149 ng/mL) at 2.8 ± 1.4 months (median, 2; range, 2 - 8 months) postoperatively.

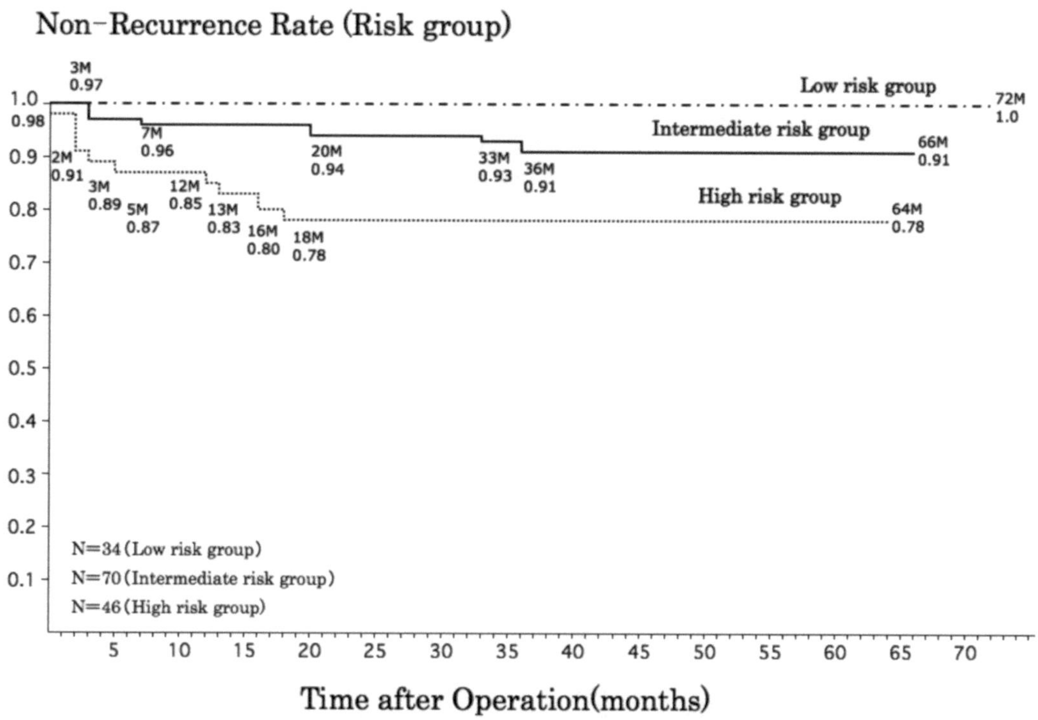

Fig. 4. Actuarial biological non-recurrence rate of each risk group

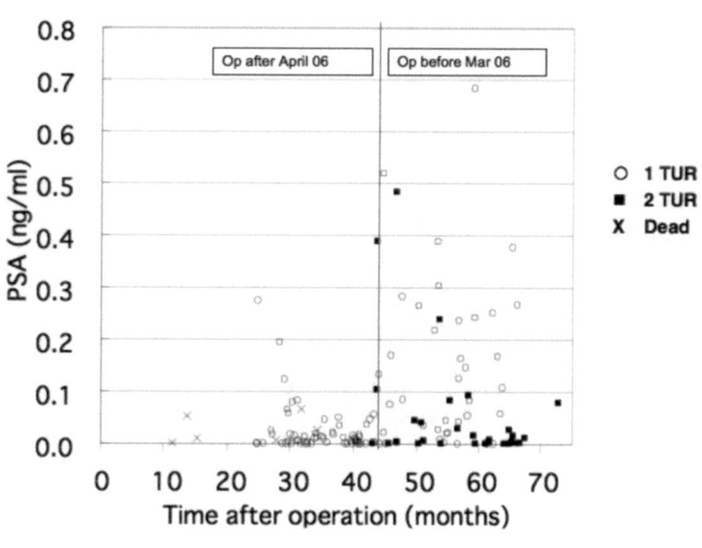

Fig. 5. Latest PSA and the time of operation

3.4 Complications

3.4.1 Urinary incontinence

We evaluated stress urinary incontinence by asking patients the postoperative status of urinary leak on a cough or a sneeze and needs for a urinary pad. Urinary incontinence was seen in 35% of the patients when a bag catheter was removed on the third postoperative day. Incontinence soon improved until the third postoperative week, and no patients need a urinary pad at all at the third postoperative month.

3.4.2 Other postoperative complications

There were no patients in whom water intoxication developed or who needed transfusions perioperatively. Bladder neck contracture, which developed three to four months postoperatively, was the most frequent complication (49 cases, 32.7%). Other complications included pubic osteitis (2 cases), bladder tamponade (2 case), acute epididymitis (3 case), pulmonary embolism (1 case), and rectourethral fistula (1 case). Erectile function was preserved after the first operation in 26 (60.5%) of the evaluated 38 sexually active patients. After the second operation only 1 out of 9 patients preserved erectile function probably due to the injury of the neurovascular bundle by excessive resection and fulguration during TUR-PCa.

Figure 6 shows an urethrocystogram 3 weeks after the operation. The seminal vesicle is clearly visualized with no extravasation from the prostate bed. Marked expansion of the prostate bed may indicate that most prostate tissues were removed by the procedure.

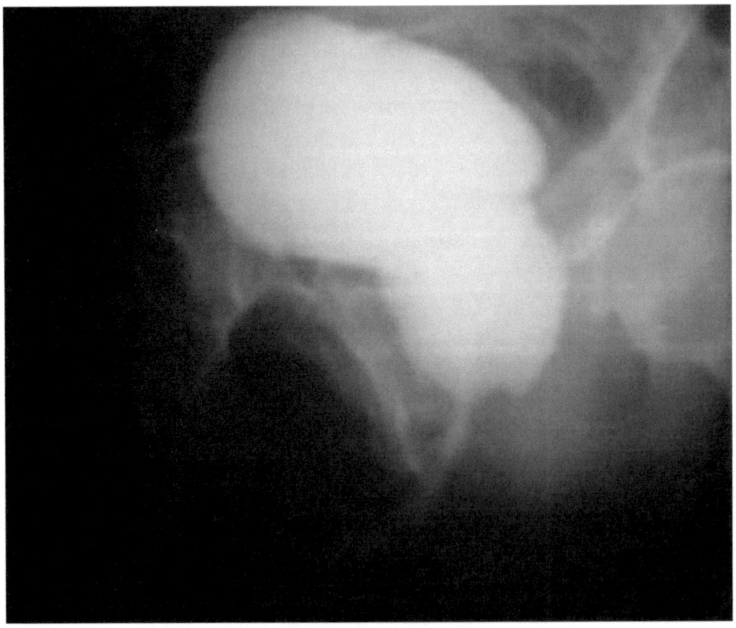

Fig. 6. Postoperative urethrocystogram (left anterior oblique)

3.5 Focal TUR-PCa: Report of a case

A 78-year–old man, who had a history of acute myocardial infarction and cerebral infarction and was on anticoagulation therapy, visited our clinic with a complaint of frequency with urge incontinence. An estimated prostate volume was 33.0 cm^3 by transrectal ultrasonography (TRUS). We started the treatment by giving alpha-blocker. His PSA at first visit was 4.20 ng/mL, and became slightly elevated to 5.47 ng/mL after two months. Transrectal prostate biopsy revealed prostate cancer confined in the right lobe. Gleason scores were 6 (3 + 3) in two out of 14 cores. He underwent standard TURP of the transition and central zone, and then we made a deeper resection of the peripheral zone of the right lobe. The operation took 80 minutes with no blood transfusion and water intoxication, and the resected weight was 27.0 g. A bag catheter was removed on the third postoperative day. The patient complained of mild dysuria that improved after two weeks, but did not complained of urinary incontinence. His erectile function had been lost preoperatively. Pathological examination confirmed prostate adenocarcinoma of Gleason score of 6 (3 + 3) in the right lobe. PSA values measured every two months were stable between 0.04 and 0.09 ng/mL till 48 postoperative weeks. The PSA values indicate the efficacy of focal TUR-PCa though final evaluation of the treatment in this patient must need longer time.

4. Discussions

4.1 Radical TUR-PCa

4.1.1 Results and complications

Transurethral resection of the prostate is now ranked as a palliative therapy used mainly to relieve obstruction caused by prostate cancer. We advanced the transurethral technique and applied it to the complete ablation of prostate tissue (RTUR-PCa). Five and 10-year biochemical recurrence-free survival rates of radical prostatectomy are reported 70-84% (M. Han et al., 2003; Zincke et al., 1994; Catalona & Smith, 1994) and 52-82% (M. Han et al., 2003; Zincke et al., 1994; Catalona & Smith, 1994; Hull et al., 2002; Pound, 1997; Roehl, et al., 2004) respectively. Our result is comparable with that of radical prostatectomy, though the number of patients and the follow-up period are not sufficient to evaluate the procedure finally at this time.

The operative technique may be more difficult than that of the standard TURP and needs more experience to become proficient. Extravasation of irrigation fluid is sure to occur during the operation, but no patients experienced water intoxication with the lowest irrigation pressure, and no patients needed blood transfusion. These suggest that the procedure can be performed safely. But much safer operation may be possible with the use of a bipolar TUR system. The postoperative course is usually uneventful and all patients could void immediately after the removal of indwelling catheters on the third postoperative day. Urinary incontinence was temporary, disappearing within 3 months. By the transurethral technique, continence can be reserved because the operator can easily detect the external sphincter, and supporting structures surrounding the prostate therefore allow the urethra to remain intact. The most excellent results of postoperative continence after radical prostatectomy are reported 93.0 % as to open prostatectomy (Walsh et al., 2000), 97.4 % as to laparoscopic surgery (Christopher et al., 2011) and 98.0 % as to robot-assisted surgery (Patel et al., 2005). And there seems no difference among the procedures when a surgeon becomes proficient. In the present study, the most frequent postoperative complication was bladder neck contracture, which had been expected because of an aggressive bladder neck resection to achieve radicality. But bladder neck contracture was easily treated by neck incision using an optical urethrotome under caudal block on a day surgery basis.

Dissemination of cancer cells may occur and affect the prognosis of patients. But the impact of TURP on the clinical outcome in patients with PCa is controversial (Levine et al., 1986; Zelefsky et al., 1993; Pansadoro et al., 1991). One report concludes that extensive TURP did not worsen the prognosis of patients with PCa (Trygg et al., 1998).
The effect of chlormadinone acetate on postoperative PSA must be considered in the present study. We could not find any reports that describe the duration of the suppressive effect of chlormadinone acetate in patients with prostate cancer. But in patients with prostate hyperplasia given 50 mg/day of chlormadinone acetate for 16 weeks, PSA levels are reported to return to the baseline levels 16 weeks after discontinuation (Noguchi et al., 2000). In this study the effect of preoperative hormonal therapy on the most recent PSA levels, therefore, can be minimum and negligible.

4.1.2 PSA failure and the second RTUR-PCa

In open or laparoscopic radical prostatectomy, residual cancer relates with PSA failure. RTUR-PCa is probably less invasive than radical prostatectomy and more flexible in the point that the second operation can be indicated and easily done to eliminate residual cancer when PSA shows a successive rise. The second RTUR-PCa was required in 46 patients. But this is considered just a technical issue because the need for the second operation has decreased as the surgeon has become experienced. There were no malignancies reported by pathologists in 13 out of 46 cases, although it is not clear whether cancer did not actually exist or missed to be detected in the specimens of the second operation. PSA failure is usually defined as a progressive rise over 0.2 ng/mL (Schild et al., 1996; Pound et al., 1999; Freedland et al., 2003). We took a careful watching policy if PSA level reached a plateau between 0.2 and 1.0 ng/mL, not regarding as PSA failure. But the second RTUR-PCa must be considered and easily performed when PSA levels start to rise continuously after the first operation.

4.1.3 Some considerations to reduce urinary incontinence and erectile dysfunction

We were able to obtain satisfactory postoperative PSA levels by RTUR-PCa comparable with open radical prostatectomy. But we recently started to think that, after a considerable number of the procedures, minimal residual prostate tissue at the part where cancer was not detected by biopsy might not necessarily prevent the radicality of the disease in carefully selected patients. We performed prostate biopsy to get information about the localization of cancer. The results of cancer localization from operative specimens were consistent with those from biopsy specimens in 46.7%. Information about the localization of cancer from biopsy specimens is very helpful to plan the manner of resection. Although an experienced resectionist can remove almost all prostate tissues transurethrally, aggressive resection can be applied where the cancer was detected by biopsy to achieve the radicality of the operation. Erectile function was preserved in about 60% of the patients in the present study. Preservation of the cavernous nerve can be achieved by leaving some prostate tissue not to be resected around the 4 or 8 o'clock position not to injure the nerve. When PSA levels rise postoperatively, removal of residual prostate tissue is possible by the second RTUR-PCa. Because the open radical prostatectomy is likely to damage the supporting tissue around the prostate and the urethra, improvement of urinary incontinence and erectile function after the operation remains limited (Stanford et al., 2000). RTUR-PCa, therefore, can provide urinary continence at least to the same degree as TURP for BPH. RTUR-PCa may be also a breakthrough to prevent the development of erectile dysfunction.

4.2 Focal TUR-PCa

4.2.1 The idea of focal therapy for prostate cancer

Currently, the two main options for the radical treatment of localized prostate cancer are radical prostatectomy (Memmelaar, 1949; Reiner & Walsh, 1979; Walsh & Donker, 1982 ; Schuessler et al., 1997; Abbou et al., 2000; Guillonneau et al., 2003 ; Binder & Kramer, 2001; Menon et al., 2002; Menon et al., 2004) and irradiation therapy (Zelefsky et al., 2002; Wahlgren et al., 2007), but post-treatment morbidities that annoy the patients include urinary incontinence and erectile dysfunction as to operative therapy, and urinary frequency, difficult urination, erectile dysfunction and rectal hemorrhage as to irradiation therapy. On the other hand, active surveillance policy or watchful waiting, which is an ultimate non-invasive procedure, is also accepted to care for the patients with low risk cancer (Bill-Axelson et al., 2008; Wilt et al., 2009). But active surveillance seems still difficult in the point to select a suitable patient, and the patient may feel anxiety about cancer progression.

4.2.2 Current options of focal therapy

Recently introduced concept of focal ablative therapy (Moul et al., 2009; Polascik et al., 2008; Eggener et al., 2007) based on the accumulated pathological and clinical findings after radical prostatectomy, may be the third idea to treat patients with localized prostate cancer. Focal therapy may contribute to minimize morbidities such as incontinence or erectile dysfunction by trying to destruct minimum prostate tissues with cancer in it. The reported rate of postoperative urinary incontinence decreased as the improvement of equipment and technique as follows: 1 to 3 % in cryotherapy (Long et al., 1998; K.R. Han et al., 2003; Hubosky et al., 2007; Polascik et al., 2007; Dhar et al., 2010) and 0.8 % in HIFU (Uchida et al., 2009).
The procedures are less invasive and repeatable, and other radical procedures can be applied when necessary after the focal therapy. One of the most important points at issue concerning the focal therapy lies in the selection of the most suitable candidate. Prostate cancer is often multifocal, and then the location of cancer must be properly diagnosed preoperatively. Because current imaging technique cannot detect a tiny focus of cancer, mapping biopsy technique is reported using a template (Onik & Barzell, 2008; Crawford et al., 2005; Furuno et al., 2004) to get information about the precise location of cancer focuses.
Procedures of focal therapy, such as cryotherapy (Onik et al., 1993; Cohen et al., 1995; Zisman et al., 2001; Babaian et al., 2008) and high intensity focused ultrasound (HIFU) (Madersbacher et al., 1995; Thüroff et al., 2003; Poissonnier et al., 2007; Lee et al., 2006), are now still thought to be an experimental one in the point that the evaluation of the efficacy is still controversial because the standard of evaluation using PSA has not been established yet. The other serious drawback of these procedures is that we cannot obtain prostate tissues. The pathological evaluation is limited only to biopsy specimens, which may confuse the results to evaluate the procedure because pathological diagnosis by operation specimen is sometimes different from that by biopsy specimen.

4.2.3 Advantages of transurethral resection

We think transurethral resection as a focal therapy for localized prostate cancer has advantages over cryotherapy or HIHU. We can control the resection of prostate tissues precisely under direct vision. We can also obtain specimens for pathological examination. PSA is applied to the follow-up examination and there remains a possibility to carry out the second TUR to aim at the radical treatment in case of PSA failure. In a patient with prostate cancer confined to one lateral lobe by biopsy, aggressive resection and fulguration can be done in the affected lobe, and appropriate non-radical resection can be applied in the other lobe only to check for cancer tissues (Morita & Matsuura, 2011). Control of prostate cancer, as a result, may be possible preserving urinary continence and erectile function.

5. Conclusion

Recent introduction of PSA into the health check up program in Japan resulted in a marked increase of patients with early stage prostate cancer. These patients were treated until now by open or laparoscopic prostatectomy, irradiation therapy including external beam irradiation and brachytherapy, hormonal therapy, watchful waiting and high intensity focused ultrasound. From the present study with the longest follow-up patients of 6 years, RTUR-PCa can be an effective treatment option for the radical treatment of prostate cancer, although the results of much longer follow up with more cases remain to be studied.

To avoid the possibility of overdiagnosis and/or overtreatment, less invasive focal TUR-PCa, can be also a suitable option of focal ablative therapy with less postoperative morbidity in carefully selected patients.

6. References

AUA Practice Guidelines Committee. (2003). AUA guideline of management of benign prostatic hyperplasia (2003). Chapter 1: Diagnosis and treatment recommendations. *Journal of Urology*, Vol.170, No.8, pp. 530-547.

Abbou, C. C., Salmon, L., Hoznek, A. et al. (2000). Laparoscopic radical prostatectomy: preliminary results. *Urology*, Vol.55, No.5, pp. 630-634.

Babaian, R. J., Donnelly, B., Bahn, D. et al. (2008). Best practice statement on cryosurgery for the treatment of localized prostate cancer, *Journal of Urology*, Vol.180, No.5, pp. 1993-2004.

Bill-Axelson, A., Holmberg, L., Filén, F. et al. (2008). Radical prostatectomy versus watchful waiting in localized prostate cancer: the Scandinavian prostate cancer group-4 randomized trial. *Journal of the National Cancer Institute*, Vol.100, No.16. pp. 1144-1154.

Binder, J. & Kramer, W. (2001). Robotically-assisted laparoscopic radical prostatectomy, *British Journal of Urology International*, Vol.87, No.4, pp. 408-410, 2001.

Catalona, W. J. & Smith, D. S. (1994). 5-year tumor recurrence rates after anatomical radical retropubic prostatectomy for prostate cancer. *Journal of Urology*, Vol.152, No.5, pp. 1837-1842.

Christopher, G., Eden, C. G., Arora, A., Hutton, A. (2011). Cancer control, continence, and potency after laparoscopic radical prostatectomy beyond the learning and discovery curves. *Journal of Endourology*, Vol.25, No.5, pp. 815-819.

Cohen, J. K., Miller R. J., Shuman, B. A. (1995). Urethral warming catheter for use during cryoablation of the prostate, *Urology*, Vol.45, No.5, pp. 861-864.

Crawford, E. D., Wilson, S. S., Torkko, K. C. et al. (2005). Clinical staging of prostate cancer: a computer-simulated study of transperineal prostate biopsy, *British Journal of Urology International*, Vol.96, No.7, pp. 999-1004.

D'Amico, A. V., Whittington, R., Malkowicz, S. B., et al. (1998). Biochemical outcome after radical prostatectomy, external beam radiation therapy, or interstitial radiation therapy for clinically localized prostate cancer. *JAMA*, Vol.280, No.11, pp. 969-974.

Dhar, N., Cher, M., Liss, Z. et al. (2010). Primary full gland and salvage prostate cryoablation: updated results from 4693 patients tracked with the cold registry, *Journal of Urology*, Vol.183, article No. e184.

Eggener, S.E., Scardino, P.T., Carroll, P.R. et al. (2007). Focal therapy for localized prostate cancer: a critical appraisal of rationale and modalities. *Journal of Urology*, Vol.178, No.6, pp. 2260-2267.

Freedland, S. J., Sutter, M. E., Dorey, F., Aronson, W. J. (2003). Defining the ideal cutpoint for determining PSA recurrence after radical prostatectomy. *Urology*, Vol.61, No.2, pp. 365-369.

Furuno, T., Demura, T., Kaneta, T. et al. (2004). Difference of cancer core distribution between first and repeat biopsy: in patients diagnosed by extensive transperineal ultrasound guided template prostate biopsy, *Prostate*, Vol.58, No.1, pp. 76-81.

Guillonneau, B., EL-Fettouh, H., Baumert, H. et al. (2003). Laparoscopic radical prostatectomy: oncological evaluation after 1000 cases at Montsouris Institute. *Journal of Urology*, Vol.169, No.4, pp. 1261-1266.

Han, K. R., Cohen, J. K., Miller, R. J. et al. (2003). Treatment of organ confined prostate cancer with third generation cryosurgery: preliminary multicenter experience, *Journal of Urology*, Vol.170, No.4, pp. 1126-1130.

Han, M., Partin, A. W., Zahurak, M. et al. (2003). Biochemical (prostate specific antigen) recurrence probability following radical prostatectomy for clinically localized prostate cancer. *Journal of Urology*, Vol.169, No.2, pp. 517-523.

Holtgrewe., H. L., Mebust., W. K., Dowd, J. B. et al. (1989). Transurethral prostatectomy: practical aspects of the dominant operation in American Urology. *Journal of Urology*, Vol.41, No.2, pp. 248-253.

Hubosky, S. G., Fabrizio, M. D., Schellhammer, P. F. et al. (2007). Single center experience with third-generation cryosurgery for management of organ-confined prostate cancer: critical evaluation of short-term outcomes, complications, and patient quality of life, *Journal of Endourology*, Vol.21, No.12, pp. 1521-1531.

Hull, G. W., Rabbani, F., Abbas, F. et al. (2002). Cancer control with radical prostatectomy alone in 1,000 consecutive patients. *Journal of Urology*, Vol.167, No.2, pp. 528-534.

Kaiho, Y., Nakagawa, H., Ikeda, Y, et al. (2005). Intraoperative electrophysiological confirmation of urinary continence after radical prostatectomy. *Journal of Urology*, Vol.173, No.4, pp. 1139-1142.

Lee, H. M., Hong, J. H., Choi, H. Y. (2006). High-intensity focused ultrasound therapy for clinically localized prostate cancer, *Prostate Cancer and Prostatic Diseases*, Vol.9, No.4, pp. 439-443.

Lepor, H., Kaci, L., Xue, X. (2004). Continence following radical retropubic prostatectomy using self-reporting instruments. *Journal of Urology*. Vol.171, No.3, pp. 1212-1215.

Levine, E. S., Cisek, V. J., Mulvihill, M. N., Cohen, E. L. (1986). Role of transurethral resection in dissemination of cancer of prostate. *Urology*, Vol.28, No.3, pp.179–183.

Long, J. P., Fallick, M. L., LaRock, D. R., Rand, W. (1998). Preliminary outcomes following cryosurgical ablation of the prostate in patients with clinically localized prostate carcinoma, *Journal of Urology*, Vol.159, No.2, pp. 477-484.

Madersbacher, S., Pedevilla, M., Vingers, L. et al. (1995). Effect of high-intensity focused ultrasound on human prostate cancer in vivo, *Cancer Research*, Vol.55, No.15, pp. 3346-3351.

Memmelaar, J. (1949). Total prostatovesiculectomy: retropubic approach. *Journal of Urology*, Vol.62, No.3, pp. 340-348.

Menon, M., Shrivastava, A., Tewari, A. et al. (2002). Laparoscopic and robot assisted radical prostatectomy: establishment of a structured program and preliminary analysis of outcomes, *Journal of Urology*, Vol.168, No.3, pp. 945-949.

Menon, M., Tewari, A., Peaboby, J. O. et al. (2004). Vattikuti Institute prostatectomy, a technique of robotic radical prostatectomy for management of localized carcinoma of the prostate: experience of over 1100 cases, *Urologic Clinics of North America*, Vol.31, No.4, pp. 701-717.

Menon, M., Shrivastava, A., Kaul, S. et al. (2007). Vattikuti Institute prostatectomy: contemporary technique and analysis of results, *European Urology*, Vol.51, No.3, pp. 648-658.

Morita, M. & Matsuura, T. (2009). Radical treatment of localized prostate cancer by radical transurethral resection of the prostate. *Current Urology*, Vol.3, No.2, pp. 87-93.

Morita, M. & Matsuura, T. (2011). An advanced but traditional technique of transurethral resection of the prostate not to overlook stage T1 prostate cancer. Current Urology, accepted for publication.

Moul, J. W., Mouraviev, V., Sun, L. et al. (2009). Prostate cancer: the new landscape. *Current Opinion in Urology*, Vol.19, No.2, pp. 154-160.

Namiki, S., Ishidoya, S., Ito, A. et al. (2009). Quality of life after radical prostatectomy in Japanese men: a 5-Year follow up study. *International Journal of Urology*, Vol.16, No.1, pp. 75-81.

Noguchi, K., Uemura, H., Takeda, M. et al. (2000). Rebound of prostate specific antigen after discontinuation of antiandrogen therapy for benign prostatic hyperplasia. *Acta Urologica Japonica*, Vol.46, No.9, pp. 605-607. (In Japanese with English summary.)

Oesterling, J. E. (1991). Prostate specific antigen: a critical assessment of the most useful tumor maker for adenocarcinoma of the prostate. *Journal of Urology*, Vol.145, No.3, pp. 907-923.

Oesterling, J. E. (1993). Using PSA to eliminate the staging radionuclide bone scan. Significant economic implications. *Urologic Clinics of North America*, Vol.20, No.4, pp. 705-711.

Onik, G. M., Cohen, J. K., Reyes, G. D. et al. (1993). Transrectal ultrasound-guided percutaneous radical cryosurgical ablation of the prostate, *Cancer*, Vol.72, No.4, pp. 1291-1299.

Onik, G. & Barzell, W. (2008). Transperineal 3D mapping biopsy of the prostate: an essential tool in selecting patients for focal prostate cancer therapy, *Urologic Oncology*, Vol.26, No.5, pp. 506-510.

Pansadoro, V., Sternberg, C. N., DePaula, F. et al. (1991). Transurethral resection of the prostate and metastatic prostate cancer. *Cancer*, Vol.68, No.8, pp. 1895-1898.

Partin, A. W., Yoo, J., Carter, H. B. et al. (1993). The use of prostate specific antigen, clinical stage and Gleason score to predict pathological stage in men with localized prostate cancer. *Journal of Urology*, Vol.150, No.1, pp. 110-114.

Patel, V. R., Tully, A. S., Holmes, R., Lindsay, J. (2005). Robotic radical prostatectomy in the community setting - the learning curve and beyond: Initial 200 cases. *Journal of Urology*, Vol.174, No.1, pp. 269-272.

Patel, V. R., Coelho, R. F., Palmer, K. J., Rocco, B. (2009). Periurethral suspension stitch during robot-assisted laparoscopic radical prostatectomy: Description of the technique and continence outcomes. *European Urology*, Vol.56, No.3, pp. 472-478.

Poissonnier, L., Chapelon, J. Y., Rouviere, O. et al. (2007). Control of prostate cancer by transrectal HIFU in 227 patients. *European Urology*, Vol.51, No.2, pp. 381-387.

Polascik, T. J., Nosnik, I., Mayes, J. M., Mouraviev, V. (2007). Short-term cancer control after primary cryosurgical ablation for clinically localized prostate cancer using third-generation cryotechnology, *Urology*, Vol.70, No.1, pp. 117-121.

Polascik, T.J., Mayes, J.M., Sun, L. et al. (2008). Pathologic stage T2a and T2b prostate cancer in the recent prostate-specific antigen era: implications for unilateral ablative therapy. *Prostate*, Vol.68, No.13, pp. 1380-1386.

Poon, M., Ruckle, H., Bamshad, R. B. et al. (2000). Radical retropubic prostatectomy: bladder neck preservation versus reconstruction. *Journal of Urology*, Vol.163, No.1, pp. 194-198.

Pound, C. R., Partin, A. W., Epstein, J. I., Walsh, P. C. (1997). Prostate-specific antigen after anatomic radical retropubic prostatectomy. Patterns of recurrence and cancer control. *Urologic Clinics of North America*, Vol.24, No.2, pp. 395-406.

Pound, C. R., Partin, A. W., Eisenberger, M. A. et al. (1999). Natural history of progression after PSA elevation following radical prostatectomy. *JAMA*, Vol.281, No.17, pp. 1591-1597.

Reiner, W. G. & Walsh, P. C. (1979). An anatomical approach to the surgical management of the dorsal vein and Santorini's plexus during radical retropubic surgery. *Journal of Urology*, Vol.121, No.2, pp. 198-200.

Reuter, M. A., Reuter, H. J., Epple, W. (1991). Total transurethral electroresection of carcinoma of the prostate. *Archivos españoles de urología*, Vol.44, No.5, pp. 611-614.

Reuter, M. A., Corredera, M., Epple, W. et al. (2008). Transurethral resection in prostate cancer, a radical procedure. Experience with 1017 cases. *Archivos españoles de urología*, Vol.61, No.1, pp. 13-26.

Rocco, B., Gregori, A., Stener, S. et al. (2007). Posterior reconstruction of the rhabdosphincter allows a rapid recovery of continence after transperitoneal videolaparoscopic radical prostatectomy. *European urology*, Vol.51, No.4, pp. 996-1003.

Roehl, K. A., Han, M., Ramos, C. G. et al. (2004). Cancer progression and survival rates following anatomical radical retropubic prostatectomy in 3,478 consecutive patients: long-term results. *Journal of Urology*, Vol.172, No.3, pp. 910-914.

Schild, S. E., Wong, W. W., Novicki, D. E. et al (1996). Detection of residual prostate cancer after radical prostatectomy with the Abbott IMx PSA assay. *Urology*, Vol.47, No.6, pp. 878-881.

Schuessler, W. W., Schlam, P. G., Clayman, R. V. et al. (1997). Laparoscopic radical prostatectomy: initial short-term experience. *Urology*, Vol.50, No. 6, pp. 854-857.

Stanford, J. L., Feng, Z., Hamilton, A. S. et al. (2000). Urinary and sexual function after radical prostatectomy for clinically localized prostate cancer: The Prostate Cancer Outcomes Study. *JAMA*, Vol.283, No.3, pp. 354-360.

Thüroff, S., Chaussy, C., Vallancien, G. et al. (2003). High-intensity focused ultrasound and localized prostate cancer: efficacy results from the European multicentric study, *Journal of Endourology*, Vol.17, No.8, pp. 673-677.

Trygg, G., Ekengren, J., Farahmand, B. Y. et al. (1998). Operative course of transurethral resection of the prostate and progression of prostate cancer. *Urologia Internationalis*, Vol.60, No.3, pp. 169-174.

Uchida, T., Shoji, S., Nakano, M. et al. (2009). Transrectal high-intensity focused ultrasound for the treatment of localized prostate cancer: eight-year experience, *International Journal of Urology*, Vol.16, No.11, pp. 881-886.

Valdivia Uría, J. G. & López López, J. A. (1989). Is the use of transurethral resection adequate in the therapy of carcinoma of the prostate? *Archivos Españoles de Urología*, Vol.42, Suppl 2, pp. 179-186.

Wahlgren, T., Nilsson, S., Lennernäs, B., Brandberg, Y. (2007). Promising long-term health-related quality of life after high-dose-rate brachytherapy boost for localized prostate cancer. *Int J Radiat Oncol Biol Phys*, Vol.69, No.3, pp. 662-670.

Walsh, P. C. & Donker, P. J. (1982). Impotence following radical prostatectomy: insight into etiology and prevention. *Journal of Urology*, Vol.128, No.3, pp. 492-497.

Walsh, P. C., Marschke, P., Ricker, D., Burnett, A. L. (2000). Patient-reported urinary continence and sexual function after anatomic radical prostatectomy. *Urology*, Vol.55, No.1, pp. 58-61.

Wilt, T. J., Brawer, M. K., Barry, M. J. et al. (2009). The Prostate cancer Intervention Versus Observation Trial: VA/NCI/AHRQ Cooperative Studies Program #407 (PIVOT): design and baseline results of a randomized controlled trial comparing radical prostatectomy to watchful waiting for men with clinically localized prostate cancer. *Contemporary Clinical Trials*, Vol.30, No.1, pp. 81-87.

Zelefsky, M. J., Whitmore, W. F. Jr., Leibel, S. A. et al. (1993). Impact of transurethral resection on the long-term outcome of patients with prostatic carcinoma. *Journal of Urology*, Vol.150, No.6, pp. 1860-1864.

Zelefsky, M. J., Fuks, Z., Hunt, M. et al. (2002). High-dose intensity modulated radiation therapy for prostate cancer: early toxicity and biochemical outcome in 772 patients. *Int J Radiat Oncol Biol Phys*, Vol.53, No.5, pp. 1111-1116.

Zincke, H., Oesterling, J. E., Blute, M. L. et al. (1994). Long-term (15 years) results after radical prostatectomy for clinically localized (stage T2c or lower) prostate cancer. *Journal of Urology*, Vol.152, No.5, pp. 1850-1857.

Zisman, A., Pantuck, A. J., Cohen, J. K., Belldegrun, A. S. (2001). Prostate cryoablation using direct transperineal placement of ultrathin probes through a 17-gauge brachytherapy template—technique and preliminary results, *Urology*, Vol.58, No.6, pp. 988-993.

3

Future Aspects of Prostate Biopsy – The Use of Primary Circulating Prostate Cells to Select Patients for Prostate Biopsy: Evidence, Utility and Cost-Benefit

Nigel P. Murray[1,2,3], Eduardo Reyes[3], Nelson Orellana[3], Ricardo Dueñas[3], Cinthia Fuentealba[3] and Leonardo Badinez[4]

[1]*Faculty of Medicine Universidad Diego Portales Santiago*
[2]*Instituto de Bio-Oncología, Santiago*
[3]*Hospital de Carabineros de Chile, Santiago*
[4]*Fundación Oncológico Arturo Pérez López, Santiago*
Chile

1. Introduction

Serum prostate specific antigen (PSA) is the only biomarker routinely used for the early detection of prostate cancer, but it is not a perfect test. Although PSA is highly specific for prostate, an elevated level is not specific for cancer, being increased in benign hyperplasia and prostatitis (Pungalia, 2006; Bozeman, 2002). Consequently, the majority of men with an increased serum PSA do not have prostate cancer and thus undergo unnecessary prostate biopsies.

Data from the USA estimate that of the million prostate biopsies performed annually, only 235,000 cases of cancer are detected, or that more than 750,000 men underwent a biopsy based on an elevated PSA caused by benign disease (Fadore, 2004; Jemal, 2006). Published data from the Prostate Cancer Prevention Trail showed that there is no cut-off point for serum PSA; for values up to 4ng/ml the sensibility of the test showed a variation of between 21% and 83%, a specificity of between 39% to 94%, with a positive predictive value of between 7% and 27% (Thompson, 2005).

2. Current indications for a prostate biopsy and the use of serum PSA

2.1 Controversies about what level of serum PSA should indicate a biopsy

At present the indications for a prostate biopsy are an abnormal digital rectal examination (DRE) and /or an increased serum PSA. However, the sensibility and specificity varies with race and the cut-off point used to indicate a biopsy. In the Finnish population, using a cut-off point of 3ng/ml and 4ng/ml the sensibility was 89% and 87% respectively (Auvienen, 2004), in Russia using a cutoff point of 4ng/ml the sensibility and specificity were 92% and 63% respectively (Matveev, 2006), while in the United States the values were 90% and 73% respectively (Labrie, 1992). Although a PSA level of 4 ng/ml is used as a cut-off point, 22%

of men with a PSA level of between 2.5 and 4.0 ng/ml have been shown to have clinically significant organ confined prostate cancer (Catalona, 1997; Horninger, 2004; Thompson, 2004). Or in other words, 62% of men with prostate cancer have a serum PSA >4.0ng/ml y 70% of all men with a serum PSA >4.0ng/ml do not have prostate cancer.

2.2 False positive rate of serum PSA and implications: Costs, increased follow-up, collateral effects of unnecessary prostate biopsies (including direct, sepsis, hemorrhage y indirect anxiety, increased follow-up)

Ideally a screening test should detect all clinically significant prostate cancers and not benign pathologies. It has been normal practice that men who are found to have an abnormal serum PSA level should have a prostate biopsy. For example, the UK Prostate Cancer Risk Management Programme (PCRMP) states "if your PSA is definitely raised, a prostate biopsy is required to determine whether cancer is present" The justification for performing biopsy in men with an abnormal PSA is that they are at high risk of prostate cancer. However, data from the Prostate Cancer Prevention Trial (Thompson, 2006) and Baltimore Longitudinal Study on Aging (Fang, 2001) have demonstrated that prostate cancer is also a common finding on biopsy in men with a *normal* PSA level. The data from this large study provide a strong argument against the use of an arbitrary PSA threshold to select men for prostate biopsy. The aim of prostate biopsy is not to detect each and every prostate cancer. After all, the Prostate Cancer Prevention Trial demonstrates that the majority of prostate cancers are in men with a normal PSA level. The aim of prostate biopsy is actually to detect those prostate cancers with the potential for causing harm.

It has been estimated that, of asymptomatic men in whom prostate cancer is detected by prostate biopsy following PSA measurement, around 50% (Draisma, 2003) do not require active treatment. Men with clinically insignificant prostate cancers that were destined never to cause any symptoms, or affect their life expectancy, may not benefit from knowing that they have the 'disease'. Indeed, the detection of clinically insignificant prostate cancer should be regarded as an (under-recognised) adverse effect of biopsy. In order to identify men who are most suitable for prostate biopsy, there is a need to identify a group at high risk, not just of prostate cancer, but of *significant* prostate cancer. Several large studies have analyzed the clinical characteristics associated with the finding of higher grade (usually defined as Gleason score ≥7) prostate cancer on biopsy. Factors significantly associated with high grade cancer were: PSA level, smaller prostate volume, abnormal DRE findings, age, and black African and black Caribbean ethnicity, whereas a previous negative prostate biopsy reduced this risk.

A false-positive PSA (or a PSA >4.0ng/mL) has consequences, firstly the collateral effects or complications of a prostate biopsy, the additional follow-up and possibility of a second or third biopsy. Observational studies, and theoretical considerations, suggest that re-biopsy will detect prostate cancer in some men with an initially negative prostate biopsy. These studies reported multivariate analyses of predictive factors for positive repeat biopsy but there was disagreement on which factors predict re-biopsy outcome. There is evidence, however, that the odds of high grade prostate cancer are reduced if a man has previously had a negative biopsy.(Djavan, 2000; Eggener, 2005; López-Corona, 2003; Mian, 2002; Roobal, 2006)

Using the results from the European Prostate Cancer Detection Study, there were no significant differences found in the tumor characteristics of stage and Gleason score comparing the first and second biopsy. The results have shown that with a second biopsy,

prostate cancer is detected in between 10% and 31% of cases (Yuen, 2004; López-Corona, 2006). However, there are patients with two negative biopsies who continue with a high suspicion of cancer, with a persistently elevated PSA or pre-malignant histology report such as prostate intraepithelial neoplasia grade 3 or atypical microacinar proliferation. The evidence suggests that cancers diagnosed with the third or fourth biopsy are those of low grade and volume (Djavan, 2001). The key question is how often is it justified to re-biopsy the patient that perhaps does not have a cancer that is life threatening. The diagnosis of a prostate cancer not clinically significant implies an overdiagnosis and over-treatment. However, there are no predictive factors, clinical or laboratorial that help to differentiate patients between men with clinically significant or not significant prostate cancer. At present the only factor available is the result of the prostate biopsy.
A prostate biopsy is not without its complications; Rietbergen et al (1993) in a study of 1687 patients reported an incidence of hematuria, hematospermia and fever in 23.6%, 45.3% and 4.2% of patients respectively. More severe complications requiring hospitalization occurred in 0.4% of patients. Moreover, Gallina et al (2008) analyzed the mortality at 120 days after an ultrasound guided prostate biopsy, the study realized in the years 1989-2000 included 22,175 patients and 1,778 controls, the mortality reported was 1.3% in biopsied men versus 0.3% in the control group.

2.3 Other indicators available based on serum PSA

Thus, a search for new biomarkers which could be more specific for the detection of prostate cancer is needed. The use of biomarkers such as percent free PSA (Lee, 2006), intact serum PSA (Steuber, 2002), serum pro-PSA(Lein, 2005) and kallikrein (Stephan, 2000) have shown to be useful in the detection of prostate cancer. However, although a biomarker could improve the precision of screening it is possible that in clinical practice it is not viable, for the need of fresh samples or high costs (Villanueva, 2006).
The use of PSA velocity has been suggested, an increase of more than 0.75ng/ml/year has been associated with an increased risk of prostate cancer and increased specific mortality (Carter, 1992; D´Amico, 2004; Heindenreich,2008). However, more recent studies have put in doubt the true role of PSA velocity, the European Randomized Study of Screening for Prostate Cancer demonstrated that increased PSA velocity was not associated with increased cancer risk, but was associated with higher grade cancers, defined as ≥ stage T1c and/or a Gleason score ≥7 (Roobol, 2006a).
Age and race adjusted PSA values has also been called in question, evaluating whether or not the PSA age adjusted range is sufficient to eliminate the need for a biopsy, revealed that 54% of patients who would not be biopsied using these criteria, had a high grade cancer diagnosed (Wolff, 2000). Similarly the free-PSA fraction has been called into doubt for the same cut-off value as with total serum PSA.

3. Circulating prostate cell detection

3.1 Theory of primary CPCs and experimental evidence

One possible candidate is the detection of circulating prostate cells (CPCs). In men with prostate cancer there is, at least, one subpopulation of cancer cells that disseminate early, to the neurovascular structures and then to the circulation (Moreno, 1992). The number of cells is very small and not detected by conventional tests; however these CPCs can be detected using immunocytochemistry.

PSA is not specific for prostate cancer, circulating prostate cells have been detected in cases of prostatitis.(Murray, 2010) thus PSA expressing cells detected in blood may not represent malignancy, but benign cells that have escaped into the blood due to acute inflammation of the prostate gland. P504S (methylacyl-CoA racemase) is an enzyme that is expressed in dysplastic and malignant prostate tissue but not by normal prostate cells.(Rubin, 2002; Luo,2002) . As dysplastic cells do not disseminate, those prostate cells expressing P504S in the circulation are considered to be malignant. However, P504S is not specific to the prostate; it is expressed in normal and malignant tissues, including leukocytes. For this reason the use of double immunomarcation is essential for the identification of malignant prostate cells. A malignant prostate cell being defined as one which expresses both PSA and P504S. CPCs detected in patients with prostate cancer have been shown to express PSA and P504S (Murray, 2008).

3.2 Current methods to detect CPCs: Flow cytometry, CellSearch®, mRNA-RT-PCR, traditional immunocytochemistry

It is beyond the scope of this chapter to review in detail the different methods of detection, two published papers by Paneleaukou et al (2009), and Fehm et al (2005) have extensively reviewed the pros and cons of the different detection methods. In summary, PCR methods have a high rate of false positive results, density gradient centrifugation may be associated with increased lost of circulating cells whereas immunomagnetic separation may not recognize tumor cells which do not express EpCAM and does not differentiate between malignant and benign prostate cells.

In this article we analyze a cohort of patients who participated in a study of prostate cancer detection, comparing the use of serum PSA with the detection of circulating prostate cells and the results of the prostate biopsy (used as the gold standard). The objective was to determine the diagnostic yield of using CPC detection as a sequential screening test in men with a serum PSA and/or DRE considered abnormal.

4. Methods and patients

This was a prospectively designed cohort study carried out in the Hospital de Carabineros de Chile (HOSCAR) and the Hospital de la Dirección de Previsión de Carabineros de Chile (DIPRECA), the immunocytochemistry was performed at the Instituto de Bio-Oncology, Santiago, Chile during the period January 2008 and December 2010. The study protocol and written consent form was approved by the ethical committees of all three centers and all patients signed a written consent form. The study was directed with complete conformity to the principals of the Declaration of Helsinki (together with the modifications of Tokyo, Venice and Hong Kong).

All men older than 40 years and attended at HOSCAR or DIPRECA, without a previous history of prostate cancer and fulfilled the criteria's for prostate cancer screening or a prostate biopsy were invited to participate. Biopsy criteria were; serum PSA ≥4.0ng/ml and /or digital rectal examination (DRE) abnormal. Exclusion criteria were older than 85 years and a life expectancy of less than 5 years.

There were 2 groups of men; firstly men attending outpatients, where routine prostate cancer screening was carried out, in addition to the normal PSA test, the men were offered CPC diagnostic testing. These men had no previous history of prostate cancer, and fulfilled

NCCN criteria for screening (2010). The presence or absence of CPCs was compared with the serum PSA level and age.

The second group was formed of men with a suspicion of prostate cancer based on an elevated serum PSA and/or abnormal digital rectal examination, and the blood sample taken immediately before the prostate biopsy. The presence or absence of CPCs was to be compared with the biopsy results, the Gleason score, percent of sample infiltrated with cancer, and number of positive cores. The sensitivity, specificity, positive and negative predictive values were to be calculated. In men with a false negative test the details of the cancer detected would be evaluated.

This second group was analyzed in terms of cost-benefit of using CPC diagnostic testing. In the present analysis the main outcome measure was the incremental cost-utility ratio of using the detection of CPCs as opposed to serum PSA and/or abnormal digital rectal examination to indicate the need for a prostate biopsy, which calculated the saving or additional cost of implementing a screening program based on CPC. The analysis included direct medical costs of the biopsy, direct costs of adverse events (calculated from data obtained from a study conducted in the same hospital), an estimation of indirect costs in terms of lost income, were calculated as days of work lost/average Chilean wage per day as a percentage of the patient group in active employment.

Costs of pre-biopsy tests, biopsy costs (including biopsy kit, ultrasound time, procedure cost, pathology cost, drug cost, hospital bed cost) were obtained from the Hospital Costs Unit Hospital de Carabineros de Chile and Hospital DIPRECA and based on Public Health Service (PHS) list prices in the case of Public Health Patients (FONASA) and Private Health Insurance (PHI) list prices in the case of Private Patients (Isapres). Costs for CPC detection were obtained from the Instituto de Bio-Oncology Costs Unit.

Costs for complications of the biopsy were based on local estimates derived from the Hospital Statistical Unit (Vallejos, 2003). Patients with fever, defined as >38°C were hospitalized and treated with ceftriaxone 1gm iv c/12 for 7 days and metronidazol 500mg c/8 PO for 7 days, hemorrhage was treated with tranexamic acid 500mg c/8 PO for 7 days as an outpatient. Complication rates were 2.9% infection and 0.5% severe hemorrhage. The total cost of the adverse effects was estimated by multiplying the number of biopsies by the frequency of adverse events.

In men with a false positive test for PSA, an estimation of increased follow-up costs was made, this comprised of blood tests for PSA and free PSA and evaluation by the urologist every 4 months, and an estimated 8% of these patients underwent a second biopsy within one year of the first biopsy. In men with a false positive CPC detection, the hospital protocol is repetition of the CPC test with the PSA and free PSA at 4 months and evaluation by the urologist, if the PSA value increased <1.0ng/ml and remained CPC positive a second biopsy was performed. 5 patients had a repeat biopsy.

4.1 Sample preparation

After written informed consent a 4ml blood sample was collected into EDTA (Beckinson-Vacutainer®). The sample was layered onto 2ml Histopaque 1.077® (Sigma-Aldrich) at room temperature, and the mononuclear cells obtained according to manufacturer´s instructions and finally washed 3 times in phosphate buffered saline pH 7.4 (PBS). The pellet was resuspended in 100µl of autologous plasma and 25µl used to prepare each slide (sialinzed DAKO, USA). The slides were air dried for 24 hours and finally fixed in a solution of 70% ethanol, 5% formaldehyde and 25% PBS for 5 minutes and then washed 3 times with PBS.

4.2 Immunocytochemistry

Monoclonal antibodies directed against PSA clone 28A4 (Novacastro, UK) in a concentration of 2,5µg/ml were used to detect prostate cells, and identified using a detection system based on alkaline phosphatase-antialkaline phosphatase (LSAB2 DAKO, USA) with new-fuschin as the chromogen. To permit the rapid identification of positive cells there was no counter staining with Mayer´s hematoxilin. Levisamole (DAKO, USA) was used as an inhibitor of endogenous alkaline phosphatase, with positive and negative controls. Positive samples underwent a second stage of processing, using the monoclonal antibody against P504S clone13H4 (Novocastro, UK) and a system of detection based on peroxidase (LSAB2, DAKO, USA) with Vector VIP (Vector, USA) as the chromogen. Endogenous peroxidase was inhibited (DAKO, USA).

4.3 Definition of positive samples

A CPC was defined according to the criteria of ISHAGE (Borgen, 1999) and the expression of P504S according to the Consensus of the American Association of Pathologists (Rubin, 2002). A malignant CPC was defined as a cell that expressed PSA and P504S, a benign cell could express PSA but not P504S and leucocytes could be P504S positive or negative but did not express PSA (Figure 1).

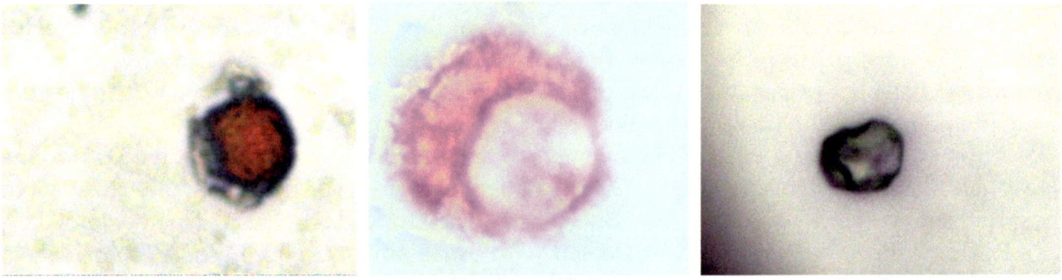

Malignant CPC **Benign CPC** **Leukocyte**

Fig. 1. Photomicrographs of the different cells type defined by immunocytochemistry.

4.4 Statistical analysis

Descriptive statistics were used for demographic variables, expressed as mean and standard deviation in the case of continuous variables with a normal distribution. In case of an asymmetrical distribution the median and inter-quartile (IQ) values were used. Noncontiguous variables were presented as frequencies. The Shapiro-Wilk test was used to determine a normal distribution. The Student T-Test was used to compare continuous variables with a normal distribution, the Mann-Whitney test for ordinate and continuous variables with a non-normal distribution and Chi-squared for the differences in frequency. For the comparison of variables between more than 2 groups the Kruksal-Wallis test was used. The diagnostic accuracy for the test detecting CPCs was analyzed using standard parameters. For this purpose patients were classified as having or not having prostate cancer. For the purpose of the use of the number of CPCs detected/ml as a diagnostic tool, and only as a mathematical exercise the number of CPCs detected/ml was considered as a continuous variable. A type I error was considered at 0.05, a type II error as 0.20 and the analysis was performed using the Stata 11.0 program.

5. Results

Group 1: 533 men with an average age of 65.1 ±9.6 years participated in the study, the relation with the detection of CPCs with the serum PSA level is shown in Table 1. There was a significant difference in the frequency of CPC detection in relation to the serum PSA level, Chi-squared for trends p<0.0001, with an odds ratio of 1.00, 2.88.5.02 and 25.60 respectively for the four groups. Comparing individually the four groups there were significant differences, except for comparing men with a serum PSA of 2.0-<3.0 with the 3.0-<4.0ng/ml group.

	Serum PSA (ng/ml)				
	<2.0ng/ml	2.0-<3.0ng/ml	3.0-<4.0ng/ml	>4.0ng/ml	Total
N° Patients	335	101	63	33	533
N° Patients CPC positive	15 (4.5%)	12 (11.9%)	12 (19.1%)	18 (55%)	57 (10.7%) p<0.0001 Chi squared for trends.
Odds ratio	1.00	2.88	5.02	25.60	

Table 1. The frequency of CPC detection according to serum PSA level

The results of comparing the frequency of CPC detection with age are shown in Table 2. There were no significant differences in the detection of CPCs between the different age groups.

Group 2: 228 men participated and underwent prostate biopsy with a mean age of 66.8±8.8 years and a median serum PSA of 5.15ng/ml (IQ 3.2)(Table 3). Of the 228 biopsies, 65 (28.6%) had adenocarcinoma of the prostate detected . CPCs were detected in 71 (31.4%) of all patients, considering men with a prostate biopsy positive for cancer, 86.15% had CPCs detected (Table 4).

	< 50 years	50-59 years	60-69 years	70-79 years	≥80 years	Total
N° Patients	28	131	214	124	36	533
N° Patients CPC positive	3 (10,7%)	14 (10.7%)	21 (9.8%)	14 (11.2%)	5 (13.9%)	57 (10.7%)
Odds ratio	1.00	0.72	0.65	0.76	0.83	p=0.98 Chi squared for trends

Table 2. The frequency of CPC detection according to age.

5.1 Association between the detection of CPCs and clinical parameters

There was no association between the detection of CPCs and age (p=0.61), but there was an association between the presence or absence of CPCs with the median PSA level (Table 4).

5.2 Association between the presence of CPCs and the detection of prostate cancer

86.2% of the patients with prostate cancer on biopsy had CPCs detected. In global terms and statistically significant, patients with cancer and CPCs detected had a higher serum PSA, a higher Gleason score and more advanced clinical stage than those with CPC negative cancer (Table 5).

N° Patients	228
Mean age (years) (SD)	66.8(8.8)
Diagnosis:	
• Cancer, % (n)	28.6 (65)
• No cancer ,% (n)	71.4(163)
PSA ng/dl, median (IQR)	5.15 (3.2)
PSA > 4 ng/ml, % (n)	80.26 (183)
CPC presentes, %(n)	31 (71)
• CPC/ml, median (IQR)	3(3)
Cancer stage, % (n)	In 63 patients.
• Stage I	26.98(17)
• Stage II	49.21 (31)
• Stage III	20.63(13)
• Stage IV	3.17 (2)
Gleason, median (IQR)	5 (2)

Table 3. General characteristics of the patients. SD: Standard deviation. IQR: Interquartile range. PSA: prostate specific antigen. CPC: Circulating prostate cells. CPC/ml: Circulating prostate cells /ml.

5.3 Diagnostic yield of CPC detection

The detection of mCPCs in this cohort correctly identified 86.2% of patients with cancer (95% CI 75.3-93.5), with a specificity of 90.8% (95% CI 85.3-94.8) (Table 6) and an exactitude of 88%. The use of a serum PSA ≥4.0ng/ml and mCPC detection did not significantly improve the discrimination between patients with or without cancer; in fact it reduced the sensitivity from 86.2 to 78.5% (CI 95% 66.5-87.7). The LR+ was 9.36 and LR- was 0.15.Using the number of mCPC detected/ml, instead of a positive-negative score, and a cutoff point of 4cells/ml only increased the specificity by 8%.

5.4 Predictive values

(Table 4) The PPV in the complete group of patients (cancer prevalence of 28.5%) was 78.9% (CI 95% 67.6-87.7) and the NPV was 94.3% (CI 95% 89.4-97.3). In the group with a serum PSA <4.0ng/ml (cancer prevalence 13.3%) the most striking result was that of the NPV of 97.1% (CI 95% 84.7-99.9), the rest of the values of predictive estimates were of low precision (Table 6).

5.5 Patients false positive

Fifteen men had a false positive result, with a mean age of 63.3±SD7.4 years and a median serum PSA of 4.36 ng/ml (IQR 2.74ng/ml). Two patients had a principal diagnosis of chronic prostatitis and 13 patients benign hyperplasia. Men with a true positive had a significantly higher frequency of a PSA >4.0ng/ml and higher number of CPCs/ml than false positive men. (Table 5)

	mCPC positive	CPC negative	p
Patients % (n)	31.14 (71)	68.86 (157)	
Mean age (SD)	66.5 (9.5)	67.0 (8.5)	0.6955 *
PSA ng/ml, median (IQR)	5.62 (4.64)	4.93 (3.08)	0.0402 **
PSA > 4ng/ml, % (n)	84.51 (60)	78.34 (123)	0.279 ***
Biopsy (i) no cancer % (n)	9.15 (13)	90.85 (129)	0.0001**
(ii) cancer	86.15 (56)	13.85 (9)	0.0001**
Gleason, median (IQR)	6 (2)	4 (0)	0.0001**

Table 4. Comparison of patients CPC positive and negative.

5.6 Patients false negative

Nine patients had a prostate biopsy positive for adenocarcinoma in the absence of CPC (Table 7), there were no significant differences between men FN and VN. Comparing men true positive with those false negative, men false negative had significantly lower Gleason scores, earlier stage disease and a discretely lower serum PSA (Table 5).

	CPCm (+) N=71			CPCm (-) N=157		
	Cancer (TP)	No cancer (FP)	p	Cancer (FN)	No cancer (TN)	p
% patients (n)	79 (56)	21 (15)	0.0000*	6 (9)	94 (148)	0.0000*
Mean age (SD)	67.1 (10.0)	64.3 (7.4)	0.2435**	68.9 (8.9)	66.9 (8.5)	0.4899**
PSA ng/ml median (IQR)	5.96 (4.20)	4.36 (2.74)	0.0567***	4.80 (0.73)	4.9 (3.15)	0.5945***
PSA>4.0ng/ml	91.1 (51)	60 (9)	0.003*	88.9 (8)	77.7 (115)	0.6257*
CmCPC median (IQR)	3.5 (3)	2 (2)	0.0000***	N/A	N/A	

TP=true positive FP=false positive FN=false negative TN=true negative IQR=interquertile range, N/A=not applicable *Chi squared **T-Test ***Mann Whitney

Table 5. Comparsion between patients mCPC positive and negative.

Total sample Serum PSA <4.0ng/ml

	Estimation punctual	CI 95%	Estimation punctual	CI 95%
Prevalence cancer	28.50%	22.7-34.8	13.30%	5.1-26.8
Sensibility	86.2%	75.3-93.5	83.30%	35.9-99.6
Specificity	90.80%	85.3-94.8	84.60%	69.5-94.1
PPV	78.9%	67.6-87.7	45.5	16.7-76.6
NPV	94.3%	89.4-97.3	97.1%	84.7-99.9
LR +	9.36	5.72-15.31	5.42	2.39-12.28
LR -	0.15	0.08-0.28	0.20	0.03-1.18

NPV negative predictive value LR+ positive likelihood ratio LR- negative likelihood ratio.

Table 6. Diagnostic yield of mCPCs. CI confidence interval, PPV positive predictive value

Patient N°	Gleason	N° positive cores	% core positive
55	4 (2+2)	1/12	4%
397	4 (2+2)	1/12	8%
421	3 (2+1)	2/12	5%, 3%
448	3 (2+1)	1/12	3%
495	3 (2+1)	1/12	3%
498	4 (2+2)	2/12	2%, 1%
499	5 (2+3)	1/12	5%
715	3 (2+1)	1/12	<1%
717	4 (2+2)	1/12	<1%

Table 7. Details of Patients with prostate cancer and CPC negative.

5.7 Patients CPC positive and prostate biopsy positive for cancer

The Gleason scores and clinical stages of the 63 men diagnosed with cancer and who were CPC positive are shown in Table 3.

6. Cost-benefit

Costs: The summary of the costs are shown in Table 8.

6.1 Prostate biopsy

6.1.1 Pre-biopsy blood tests

All patients underwent standard routine blood tests pre-biopsy, with a cost of €37 PHS and €57 PHI.

6.1.2 Drug cost
All patients had prophylaxis with ciprofloxacin 500mg c/12 and metronidazol 500mg c/8 orally for 7 days and a Fleet® enema the morning of the biopsy. Sub-total cost:€15

6.1.3 Prostate biopsy kit
All patients had to bring the biopsy kit, purchased at their own cost €62.

6.1.4 Eco-guided 12 sample prostate biopsy
Costs include ultrasound, biopsy procedure, and pathological evaluation using standard H&E technique, for a cost of €64 PHS and €102 PHI.

6.1.5 Hospital room cost
PHS €16 PHI €122

6.2 CPC cost
There is no codification in PHS or PHI costs, we took the price of an immunocytochemical analysis of one tissue as the reference price, PHS €27 and PHI €43.

	PHS	PHI
Pre-biopsy blood tests	€37	€57
Drug cost	€15	€15
Biopsy Kit	€62	€62
Prostate biopsy	€64	€102
Inpatient 1 day	€16	€122
CPC cost	€27	€43

Table 8. Costs of a prostate biopsy: PHS = public health service PHI=private health insurance

6.3 Complication cost
Costs were based on the frequency of complications requiring treatment.(table 9)

6.3.1 Sepsis
Estimated cost 228 x 2.9%= 6.61 cases. 7 days hospitalized, PHS €112 PHI €855, antibiotics 7 days €232 Total: PHS €343 PHI €1,087

6.3.2 Hemorrhage
Estimated cost, 228 x 0,5% =1.14 cases Cost outpatient: tranexemic acid 500mg c/8 for 7 days €46

6.3.3 Indirect patient costs (working days)
The average daily Chilean wage is €16, travel costs were not estimated.

6.4 Costs for total study population: 228 biopsies

The total cost of the study population of 228 patients with suspicion of prostate cancer either for DRE findings and/or PSA ≥4.0ng/ml is shown in Table 9, the estimated complication costs, include indirect costs. The total cost was divided by the 228 patients to achieve a weighted cost/biopsy.

6.5 Costs for study group using CPC detection and omitting biopsies in CPC negative patients

The total cost of 228 CPC detection tests was €6,074 (PHS) and €9,719 (PHI), with the additional cost of 71 biopsies to be carried out in CPC positive men, the total cost for each group is shown in Table 10.

	PHS outpatient	PHS inpatient	PHI outpatient	PHI inpatient
Pre-biopsy tests	€8,393	€8,393	€12,990	€12,990
Drug cost	€3,371	€3,371	€3,371	€3,371
Biopsy Kit	€14,179	€14,179	€14,179	€14,179
Biopsy	€14,533	€14,533	€23,327	€23,327
Inpatient Indirect costs	€0 €3,660	€3,633 €7,320	€0 €3,660	€27,860 €7,320
Complication costs Sepsis:(N=7) Hospitalization Antibiotics Indirect costs Hemorrhage (N=1) Drug cost Medical control Indirect costs	 €781 €1,621 €784 €45 €9 €112	 €781 €1,621 €784 €45 €9 €112	 €5,987 €1,621 €784 €45 €17 €112	 €5,987 €1,621 €784 €45 €17 €112
Total 228 patients: Per biopsy	 **€47,535** **€209**	 **€54,828** **€241**	 **€66,093** **€290**	 **€97,613** **€428**

Table 9. Cost total of 228 patients and per biopsy according to PHS, PHI in or outpatient.

6.6 Costs for study group using CPC detection and omitting biopsies in CPC negative patients

The total cost of 228 CPC detection tests was €6,074 (PHS) and €9,719 (PHI), with the additional cost of 71 biopsies to be carried out in CPC positive men, the total cost for each group is shown in Table 10.

6.7 Saving using CPC system

Table 10 shows the total cost for the normal system versus the CPC detection system and savings generated.

	Normal System	CPC System	Saving
PHS outpatient	€47,566	€20,877	€26,689
PHS inpatient	€54,828	€23,148	€31,680
PHI outpatient	€66,093	€30,300	€35,793
PHI inpatient	€97,613	€40,115	€57,498

Table 10. Total of normal system versus CPC based system and saving in 228 biopsies.

6.8 Costs of false positive tests (in the year after prostate biopsy)

Standard follow up procedure in men with an elevated PSA and biopsy negative for cancer, is a four monthly medical control with serum PSA and free serum PSA and medical control. Control procedure using CPC detection was three monthly medical control, serum PSA and CPC test. The indications for a biopsy within one year were; increase in serum PSA >1ng/ml, number of CPCs/ml increasing.

i. Standard control: serum PSA con percent free PSA: three four monthly blood tests with 3 urology consultations PHS €108 PHI €143. The number of patients in control was 163 men. The number of repeat biopsies, 8%, was estimated from patient activity records of the hospital, the number of estimated repeat biopsy was 13.
ii. CPC detection: serum PSA, CPC detection and urology consultation cost of three four monthly controls PHS €141 PHI €227. The number of patients in control was 15 and there 5 repeat biopsies.

Total cost of follow-up controls: assuming an indirect cost of half a day of work, €8/visit, for a total annual of €24.

i. Standard protocol for 163 men: PHS €21,567, PHI €40,938
ii. CPC protocol for 15 men: PHS €2,480, PHI €3,768

7. Conclusions

7.1 Patient population

The number of negative biopsies for cancer 71.49%, is similar to that reported in 2 recent studies (Schroder, 2009; Andiole, 2009). The predictive positive and negative values obtained for a serum PSA less and more than 4.0 ng/ml; and the presence of prostate cancer are similar to those previously published. In men with a DRE abnormal and serum PSA <4.0ng/ml 13.3% (6/45) had a biopsy positive for cancer of those men with a serum PSA ≥4.0ng/ml, 32.2% (59/183) had cancer detected (Misky, 2003). We conclude that our patient sample typically represents that of the general screening population.

7.2 Diagnostic yield

It is important to emphasize that the detection of CPCs was a sequential test, used in men with a high serum PSA and/or abnormal DRE, therefore a direct comparison with performance diagnosis the serum PSA is not possible. However, an earlier study (Murray, 2010) did not demonstrate a cut-off point for the detection of CPCs in relation to the serum PSA, which is important as it is estimated that approximately 42% of men with prostate cancer have a serum PSA <4.0ng/ml (Lodding, 1995) . Thus the test could be useful to identify men with a PSA <4.0 ng/ml at risk for prostate cancer.

7.2.1 Negative predictive value

Probably more important, is that the NPV of 94.3% in a sample of patients with a prevalence of cancer of 28,5% and suspicion of cancer that requires a biopsy, showed that the absence of mCPCs had a high discriminating power. This suggests that men with an increased serum PSA and/or abnormal DRE but mCPC negative could be considered of being at low risk and thus a biopsy might not be necessary. From the point of view of the -LR of 0.15, this permits the reduction of the probability of PC in almost 40% (McGee, 2002) which when applied to a prevalence of approximately 50% significantly reduces the probability of cancer post-test to around 10%. This is clinically useful when determining whether or not to continue investigating a patient. Including, if the cancer was initially missed using the mCPCs test (13.8% of cancers in the study), all the missed cancers were low grade (Gleason 3 or 4, except 1 patient with a Gleason 5 tumor. This patient underwent surgery, the surgery specimen showed a Gleason 5 tumor, infiltrating 5% of 1 lobe, without peri-neural, lymphatic, vascular or capsular invasion, the type of cancer which fulfills NCCN criteria for active surveillance (2010).

7.3 Comparison with other methods of CPC detection

The FN result obtained in this study compares with the 24.7% of mCPC negative prostate cancer reported in patients prior to radical prostatectomy and was associated with small low grade tumors and little risk of the presence of bone marrow micrometastasis (Murray, 2010a). This study used the same methodology, defining mCPCs as being P504S and PSA positive.

However, other studies of detection of circulating prostate cells, using a different methodology have been discordant results. Using a dual PSA/prostate specific membrane antigen RT-PCR method Eschwege et al (2009) only found 37% of pre-operative patients to be CPC positive. Davis et al (2008) found no association between CPC detection using the CellSearch® system and the clinical parameters prior to radical prostatectomy or between men with local PC or controls. Likewise in studies using RT-PCR with mRNA PSA no differences were found between patients with localized cancer and healthy subjects in the frequency of CPCm detection (Patel, 2004). We believe that part of this difference is the relatively high detection in control patients. One explication is that CPC can be found in men with prostatitis, however these CPCs are P504S negative (Murray, 2010). This underlies the problem with different methods used to detect circulating tumor cells.

The test using CPCs was designed with a result considered as positive or negative, the incorporation of the number of cells detected/ml increased the specificity by 8% but significantly reduced the sensibility. The CellSearch® system uses a cutoff value of 5 cells/7.5ml of blood to classify a test as positive in patients with metastasis (Davis, 2008; Resel, 2010). However, we consider that in the different stages of a cancer the information needed to make clinical decisions varies. In patients with metastatic cancer the question is one of prognosis, where a determined cutoff value could divide patients in good and bad prognosis, or the change of circulating cell numbers as a measure of response to treatment. In our study the fundamental question was "is there cancer?" Consequently we considered that the presence of single cell is sufficient to classify patients as positive or negative for cancer. Using a cutoff value of 5cells/ml the specificity was 98.77% but the sensitivity decreased to 29.3%, with the utility of the test being significantly decreased.

7.4 Application of the test to clinical practice

A prostate biopsy is not without risks to the patient, Rietbergen et al (1997), in a study of 5,802 patients undergoing transrectal prostate biopsy reported an incidence of complications of 0.5% hospitalizations, 2.1% rectal hemorrhage, 2.3% fever and 7.2% persistent hematuria. A study of 381 patients biopsied in the Hospital DIPRECA revealed that 1.57% of patients were hospitalized with fever, treatment was with 7 days of intravenous antibiotics (Vallegas, 2003).
There is an urgent need for an additional diagnostic test which could reduce costs and avoid the risks of unnecessary PB in patients at low risk of cancer; these patients could be actively followed. A persistent increase in serum PSA or the appearance of mCPCs during follow up could be an indication for a biopsy; however, this is yet to be substantiated.

7.5 Principal limitations of the study

1. The test was analyzed by one trained cytologist, and as such requires validation with different observers. However, this could be overcome with training and the results could be reproducible between different centers. Equally, the DRE and decision to carry out a biopsy is dependent on the urologist.
2. The study was designed as a sequential test, mCPC detection being requested after the serum PSA and/or DRE, forming a diagnostic test in series. Inspite of this the NPV increased, instead of decreasing as is usual in these types of studies. Although it is unknown the diagnostic yield when comparing with the serum PSA independently and blinded, for which caution is urged before considering the test for routine use, especially for screening, follow up of FN cases or as an isolated tool.
3. The study did not separately analyze the contribution of the serum PSA and/or DRE in the pre-test determination of detecting PC, for which it is unknown the contribution of each in the decision to perform a biopsy. However, this constitutes the daily practice of prostate cancer screening, for which it could be viewed as a strongpoint in demonstrating the diagnostic yield of mCPC detection in the real world.
4. The absence of follow-up of FP patients. Fifteen men had a false positive result for mCPCs, as yet the follow up data with serial serum PSA and mCPCs or a second biopsy are not available. This point is being evaluated in a follow-up study which is currently in progress.

8. Cost-analysis

There is consensus in that evidence surrounding new technologies should include cost-effectiveness information. These economic evaluations are part of the daily practice in many countries, such as the United Kingdom. In the case of Latinamerica, including Chile, Pichon-Riviere et al (2008) have shown that there is limited use of the information collected from the evaluations of health technologies, limited resources designated for their development and little government support for these initiatives. In spite of this, countries such as Brazil, Mexico, Chile and Argentina have an active policy of evaluating health technologies and it appears that this is the tendency in other countries in the region (Banta, 2009).
In the process of prioritization and selection of health interventions, included in different packets (public health, community health programs of low and intermediate complexity, special health programs and those of high complexity), the disease frequency and evaluations of cost-benefit play a fundamental role (González-Pier, 2006). Chile has a mixed public-private health system, in that the public health insurance FONASA is financed on the

basis of the social security and fiscal support which covers 70% of the population and a private health insurance system, the ISAPRES which covers a further 16% of the Chilean population (Health Ministry, Chile, 2009).

In this context, our study makes a contribution of the decision making process of incorporating new health technologies. The Chilean male population aged between 45 and 75 years, according the 2003 Census, is estimated to be in 2010 and 2015 approximately 2,296,000 and 2,618,300. Using the results of the First Health Survey of the Health Ministry in 2003, it estimates there will be 95,425 men in 2010 and 116,241 men in 2015 with a serum PSA >4,0ng/ml. However, there is no national record of the number of prostate biopsies performed on an annual basis. The number of patients diagnosed in the public health service between 2005 and 2010 with prostate cancer was 17,719, assuming a positive biopsy rate of 27%, this corresponds to approximately 14,100 biopsies/year in the public health service. This represents 14.8% of the potential population of men with a serum PSA >4.0ng/ml.

Our pilot study has shown that it is possible to eliminate 70% of first time prostate biopsies with the use of the CPC system, which translates into a saving of between €23,874 and €51,807 in the 228 patients who were studied. If the results are confirmed in a larger number of patients this would represent a saving of between €1,465,829 and €3,180,998 per year, assuming an average of 14,000 biopsies/year.

We used a simple standard manual method of CPC detection, in the market there is the FDA approved CellSearch® system for detecting CPCs. However, the costs of the test on the open market are between U$770 and US1,000. We consider that with an experienced immunocytologist the manual method and based on our results the method is acceptable. This means that the cost of installing the CPC program in terms of equipment is of zero cost, as all elements are found in a routine laboratory. The cost per test is much less, €23,50 per test, including labor costs.

Consistent with the findings of others documenting relatively high false-positive rates (Glick, 1998; Sonneberg, 2002; Mohadevia, 2003), we found a substantial number (163/228) of those undergoing cancer screening to incur at least one false-positive result, in terms of a serum PSA >4.0ng/ml. The CPC detection test had a significantly lower false positive rate (15/71). The majority of individuals who incurred a false positive screen result received some type of follow-up care in the year following their screening. Despite some individuals not receiving any follow-up care, rates of medical utilization for specific follow-up tests were almost always higher in the false-positive group. This translated into significantly more medical care costs. We calculated that men with a serum PSA >4.0ng/ml and negative first prostate biopsy incurred an average cost of PHS $90,414 and PHI $145,350. The number of men with a false positive CPC detection test is much lower, and although the cost per patient was higher, the overall cost for the system was much less, in terms of costs and medical time. We estimated the number of repeat biopsies taken in these patients from previous hospital data, which further increases costs. When false-positive findings and their consequences are explicitly considered in economic evaluations, model results are often sensitive to the assumed rate of false positive screens (Etiziona, 1995; Chirikas 2002). These results have led some to argue that the cost-effectiveness of different screening programs are primarily driven by rates of false-positive screens among other undesirable outcomes (e.g., over-diagnosis). The reality is that false-positive findings among those undergoing cancer screenings are relatively common, usually constituting the large majority of all positive findings and often leading to follow-up investigations that do not result in a cancer diagnosis (Etzioni, 1995). Given the potential economic and other implications of a false-positive cancer screen result, it is important that when patients are offered cancer screening it is within a context that allows informed decision-making.

However, despite the convincing evidence in our pilot study of 228 patients, the implementation of CPC detection might result in unanticipated losses or dis-econcomies in the short run. There are two prime reasons, firstly that the new cost-effective technology will probably co-exist with the inefficient alternative for a considerable time period. In our study the idea is a complementary process, leading to decreased biopsies, thus there is not an alternative test; only that CPC detection is not performed. Secondly there might be dis-economies of learning, during the implementation phase, old and new practices may co-exist, with most health professionals being less familiar with new technologies than with the old process. Economies of learning refer to decreasing average cost or increasing average effectiveness, as a result of accumulating experience and know-how. The transition from old to new processes may well cause the opposite effect; increasing average costs or decreasing effectiveness as experience is lacking. Thus patients may have CPC detection performed and regardless of the result proceed to prostate biopsy. The investment necessary to embed the technology in the health organization was not calculated, this would mean capacitating health professionals, information to the patient of the incorporation of new test. That this study was performed as part of a clinical trial, thus had an experimental design, the reality in the clinical situation may be different, and a focus on common practice to order to consider the impact of potentially cost-effective technology on the production processes and budgetary constraints in the health organization.

In summary, we consider that the CPC detection test has an important impact in terms of cost-benefit in the context of a prostate cancer screening program, decreasing the number of deserve to be confirmed with a larger number of patients in an environment of common screening practice.

9. Acknowledgements

To Mrs. Ana María Palazuelos de Murray for her help and patience during the project and writing of the manuscript.

10. References

Andiole GL, Grubb RL III, Buys SS, et al (2009). Mortality results from a randomized prostate cancer screening trial. NEJM 360: 1310-19.

Auvinen A, Maattanen L, Finne P, et al(2004) Test sensitivity of prostate-specific antigen in the finnish randomised prostate cancer screening trial. Int J Cancer. 111(6):940-943.

Banta D (2009). Health technology assessment in Latin America and the Caribbean. International Journal of Technology Assessment in Health Care 25: 253-2.

Borgen E, Naume B, Nesland JM, et al. (1999) Standardization of the immunocitochemical detection of cancer cells in bone marrow and blood: Establishment of objective criteria for the evaluation of immunostained cells. *ISHAGE* Cytotherapy; 5: 377-88.

Bozeman CB, Carver BS, Eastham JA, et al. (2002) Treatment of chronic prostatitis lowers serum prostate specific antigen. J Urol 167: 1723-6.

Carter HB, Pearson JD, Metter EJ, et al (1992). Longitudinal evaluation of prostate-specific antigen levels in men with and without prostate disease. JAMA. 267:2215–2222

Catalona WJ, Smith DS and Ornstein DK.(1997) Prostate cancer detection in men with serum PSA concentrations of 2.6 to 4.0 ng/ ml and benign prostate examination. Enhancement of specificity with free PSA measurements. JAMA 277: 1452-1455

Chirikos TN, Hazelton T, Tockman et al(2002). Screening for lung cancer with CT: a preliminary cost-effectiveness analysis. Chest 121:1507 - 14.

D'Amico AV, Chen MH, Roehl KA, et al(2004). Preoperative PSA velocity and the risk of death from prostate cancer after radical prostatectomy. N Engl J Med.351:125–135. Davis JW, Nakanishi H, Kumar VS, Bhadkamkar VA et al(2008). Circulating tumor cells in peripheral blood samples from patients with increased serum prostate specific antigen: initial results in early prostate cancer. J Urol. 179(6):2187-91; discussion 2191.

Draisma G, Boer R, Otto SJ, et al (2003) Journal of the National Cancer Institute, 95(12): 868–878.

Djavan B, Zlotta A, Remzi M, et al(2000). Optimal predictors of prostate cancer on repeat prostate biopsy: a prospective study of 1,051 men. J Urol, 163: 1144–1148.

Djavan B, Ravery V, Zlotta A, et al (2001). Prospective evaluation of prostate cancer detected on biopsies 1, 2, 3 and 4: when should we stop? J Urol.166:1679-1683

Eggener SE, Roehl KA & Catalona WJ (2005) . Predictors of subsequent prostate cancer in men with a prostate specific antigen of 2.6 to 4.0 ng/ml and an initially negative biopsy. J Urol, 174: 500–504.

Eschwège P, Moutereau S, Droupy S, et al(2009). Prognostic value of prostate circulating cells detection in prostate cancer patients: a prospective study. Br J Cancer. 100(4):608-10.

Etzioni R, Cha R, Cowen ME (1999). Serial prostate specific antigen screening for prostate cancer: a computer model evaluates competing strategies. J Urol 162:741 - 8.

Fadare O, Wang S, Mariappan MR (2004). Practice patterns of clinicians following isolated diagnoses of atypical small acinar proliferation on prostate biopsy specimens. Arch Pathol Lab Med 128: 557-60.

Fang J, Metter EJ, Landis P, et al (2001): Low level of prostate-specific antigen predicts long term risk of prostate cancer: results from the Baltimore Longitudinal Study on Aging. Urology 58: 411-416.

Fehm T, Sotomayer EF, Meng S, et al(2005). Methods for isolating epithelial cells and criteria for their classification as carcinoma cells. Cytotherapy 7:171-85

Gallina A, Suardi N, Montorsi F, et al(2008). Mortality at 120 days after prostatic biopsy: a population-based study of 22,175 men. Int J Cancer. 123(3):647-52

Glick S, Wagner JL, Johnson CD (1998). Cost-effectiveness of doublecontrast barium enema in screening for colorectal cancer. AJR Am J Roentgenol 170:629 - 36.

González-Pier E, Gutiérrez-Delgado C, Stevens G,et al.,. Priority setting for health interventions in Mexico's System of Social Protection in Health. Lancet 2006; 368: 1608-18.

Heidenreich A (2008). Identification of high-risk prostate cancer: role of prostate-specific antigen, PSA doubling time, and PSA velocity. Eur Urol. 54(5):976-7; discussion 978-Schroder FH,

Horninger W, Berger AP, Rogatsch H, et al(2004): Characteristics of prostate cancers detected at low PSA level. Prostate 58: 232-237.

Jemal A, Siegel R, Ward E, , et a (2006). Cancer statistics. Cancer J Clin 56: 106-30.

Labrie F, DuPont A, Suburu R, et al (1992). Serum prostate specific antigen as pre-screening test for prostate cancer. J Urol. 147:846-851.

Lee R, Localio AR, Armstrong K, et al (2006). A meta-analysis of the performance characteristics of the free prostate specific antigen test. Urology 67: 762-8.

Lein M, Semjonow A, Graefen M, et al (2005). A multicenter clinical trial of the use of (-5, -7) pro prostate specific antigen. J Urol 174: 2150-3.

Lodding P, Aus G, Bergdahl S (1998). Characteristics of screening detected prostate cancer in men 50 to 66 years old with 3-4ng/ml PSA. J Urol 159: 899-903

Lopez-Corona E, Ohori M, Scardino PT, et al(2004). A nomogram for predicting a positive repeat prostate biopsy in patients with a previous negative biopsy session.[erratum appears in J Urol. 171(1):360–1]. J Urol, 2003; 170: 1184–1188.

Lopez-Corona E, Ohori M, Wheeler TM, , et al(2006). Prostate cancer diagnosed after repeat biopsies have a favorable pathological outcome but similar recurrence rate. J Urol. 175:923-930

Luo J, Zha S, Gage WR et al (2002). Alpha-methylacyl-CoA racemase: a new molecular marker for prostate cancer. Cancer Res 62: 2220-6.

Mahadevia PJ, Fleisher LA, Frick KD, et al (2003).Lung cancer screening with helical computed tomography in older adult smokers: a decision and cost-effectiveness analysis. JAMA 289:313 - 22.

Matveev V (2006). Screening of prostate cancer. Is it Needed?. Russian experience. Arch Ital Urol Androl. 78(4):149.151

McGee S (2002). Simplifying likelihood ratios. J Gen Intern Med 17: 646-649

Mian BM, Naya Y, Okihara K, et al(2002). Predictors of cancer in repeat extended multisite prostate biopsy in men with previous negative extended multisite biopsy. Urology, 60: 836–840.

Mistry K, Cable G (2003). Meta-analysis of PSA and digital rectal examination as screening tests for prostate carcinoma. J Am Board Fam Pract 16: 95-101

Moreno JG, Croce CM, Fischer R, et al (1992). Detection of hematogenous micrometastasis in patients with prostate cancer. Cancer Res 52: 6110-6112

Murray NP, Badínez L (2008). Las células prostáticas en la circulación sanguínea en pacientes con cáncer prostático expresan la proteína P504S: un estudio utilizando inmunocitoquímica. Rev Chil Urol 73: 54-7.

Murray NP, Calaf GM, Badinez L, et al (2010). P504S expressing circulating prostate cells as a marker for prostate cancer. Oncology Reports 24: 687-692.

Murray NP, Reyes E, Badínez L, et al (2010a). Detección y características de células prostáticas circulantes primarias, asociación con la presencia de micrometástasis y las implicaciones para el tratamiento quirúrgico en hombres con cáncer prostático. Arch. Esp. Urol. 63: 345-53

NCCN Clinical Oncology Guidelines 2010. www.nccn.org

Panteleakou Z, Lembessis P. Sourla A, et al(2009). Detection of circulating tumor cells in prostate cancer patients: methodological pitfalls andclinical relevance. Mol Med 15: 101-14

Patel K, Whelan PJ, Prescott S, et al (2004). The Use of Real-Time Reverse Transcription-PCR for Prostate-Specific Antigen mRNA to Discriminate between Blood Samples from Healthy Volunteers and from Patients with Metastatic Prostate Cancer. Clin Cancer Res 10: 7511-9

Pichon-Riviere A. (2008) 'HTA in Latin-America and the Caribbean (LAC), facilitators and barriers for international collaboration: a survey'. V Annual Meeting, 9 de Julio, Montréal Canadá.

Pungalia RS, D'Amico AV, Catalona WJ, et al(2006). Impact of age, benign prostatic hyperplasia and cancer on prostate specific antigen level. Cancer 106: 1507-113

Resel L, Olivier C, San José L, et al. (2010) , Immunomagnetic quantification of circulating tumoral cells in patients with prostate cancer: clinical and pathological correlation. Arch Esp Urol. 63:23-31.

Rietbergen JB, Kruger AE, Kranse R, et al (1997). Complications of transrectal ultrasound guided systematic sextant biopsies of the prostate: evaluation of complication rates and risk factors within a population based screening program. Urology 49: 875-80.

Roobol MJ, Schroder FH, Kranse R & ERSPC R (2006). A comparison of first and repeat (four years later) prostate cancer screening in a randomized cohort of a symptomatic men aged 55–75 years using a biopsy indication of 3.0 ng/ml (results of ERSPC, Rotterdam). Prostate, 66: 604–612.

Roobol MJ, van der Kwast TH, Kranse R, et al(2006a). Does PSA velocity predict prostate cancer in pre-screened populations? Eur Urol. 49:460–465. discussion 465.

Rubin MA, Zhou M, Dhanasekaran SM et al (2002). Alpha-methyl-acyl coenzyme A racemase as a tissue biomarker for prostate cancer. JAMA 287: 1662-70.

Schroder FH, Hugosson J, Roobol MJ, et al (2009). Screening and prostate cancer mortality in a randomized European Study. NEJM 360: 1320-8.

Sonnenberg A (2002). Cost-effectiveness in the prevention of colorectal cancer. Gastroenterol Clin North Am 31:1069 - 91.

Stephan C, Jung K, Lein M, et al (2000). Molecular forms of prostate specific antigen and human kallikrien 2 as promising tools for early diagnosis of prostate cancer. Cancer Epidemiol Biomarkers Prev 9: 1133-47.

Steuber T, Nurmikko P, Haese A, et al (2002). Discrimination of benign from malignant prostate disease by selective measurements of single chain, intact free prostate specific antigen. J Urol 168: 1917-22.

Superintendencia de Salud. Departamento Planeamiento Institucional-Estudios. [http://www.fonasa.cl/prontus_fonasa/site/artic/20070112/asocfile/01_demografia_pagina_web__08_06_2009_jav.xls#T1.1.1!A1]. [Acceso 17 de Enero de 2011].

Thompson IM, Pauler DK, Goodman PJ, et al (2004): Prevalence of prostate cancer among men with a prostate-specific antigen level ≤4.0 ng per millimeter. N Eng J Med 350: 2239-2246.

Thompson IM, Ankerst DP, Chi C, et al (2005). Operating characteristics of prostate specific antigen in men with an initial PSA level of 3,0ng/ml or lower. JAMA 294: 66-70.

Thompson IM, Ankerst DP, Chi C, et al(2006) . Assessing prostate cancer risk: results from the Prostate Cancer Prevention Trial.[see comment]. J Natl Cancer Inst, 98: 529–534.

Vallejos T, Gonzalez G (2003). Complicaciones en biopsia prostática transrectal ecoguiada Rev Chil Urol 68: 143-145.

Villaneuva J, Schaffer DR, Phillip J et al (2006). Differential exoprotease activities confer tumor specific serum peptidone patterns. J Clin Invest 116: 271-84.

Wolff JM, Brehmer B, Borchers H, et al(2000). Are age-specific reference ranges for prostate specific antigen population specific? Anticancer Res. 20(6D):4981-3.

Yuen JS, Lau WK, Ng LG, et al (2004). Clinical, biochemical and pathological features of initial and repeat transrectal ultrasonography prostate biopsy positive patients. Int J Urol. 11:225-231.

4

Technical Advices for Prostate Needle Biopsy Under Transrectal Ultrasound Guidance

Makoto Ohori[1] and Ayako Miyakawa[2]
[1]*Dept. of Urology, Tokyo Medical University*
[2]*Dept. of Molecular Medicine and Surgery, Unit of Urology, Karolinska Institute*
[1]*Japan*
[2]*Sweden*

1. Introduction

In the early 1990's when systematic biopsy of prostate using transrectal ultrasonography (TRUS) had just begun, there was enthusiasm for identifying abnormalities and obtaining appropriate samples. Since the occurrences of early small prostate cancer are increasing and identifying tumors using TRUS are somewhat subjective, the efficiency of the method in detecting and staging prostate cancer has decreased. (Ohori, et al. 2003) Instead, many physicians discuss about where and how many biopsy cores should be taken in order to improve the detection-rate of cancer. Clinicians have also focused on the pathological features of cancer in biopsy specimens that sometimes provide significant information to stage prostate cancer. (Satake, et al. 2010) Prostate biopsy itself is not technically challenging and residents as well as fellows are regularly in charge of the biopsy - with or without ultrasound technicians. Those with less experience of TRUS guided biopsy are helped by studying technical advices to get appropriate specimens. At Baylor College of Medicine, Memorial Sloan-Kettering Cancer Center, and Tokyo Medical University we have performed more than 5000 cases of TRUS guided prostate biopsy. This large number of TRUS guided prostate biopsies has provided several technical tips to obtain appropriate tissue samples and to avoid complications such as rectal bleeding. In this chapter we will describe practical methods that will improve prostate biopsy.

2. Direction of needle

Non-visible prostate cancer on TRUS has been increased because of the advances in PSA screening. (Ohori, et al.2003) However, there are still occurrences of hypoechoic lesions suspicious for cancer. To obtain an appropriate tissue sample from suspicious lesions, it is better to make the needle tip facing the rectum (Figure 1, 2). Otherwise, the needle tip slips away from the prostate so that it may result in inappropriate samples and missing lesions. This is particularly true when the biplane ultrasound probe is used which is close to parallel to the rectum.
When a probe with end-fire is used for a biopsy, the location of the biopsy should be close to the side of urethra (Figure 3). If a needle is located like in figure 3 (left), it may cause long distances between the tip of needle and the prostate capsule so that there is adipose tissue between them. It may cause significant bleeding. Similarly, if one prefers to do biopsy with

transverse image, the direction of the biopsy device should be as in the figure to reduce the distance between the prostate capsule and tip of the needle (Figure 4).

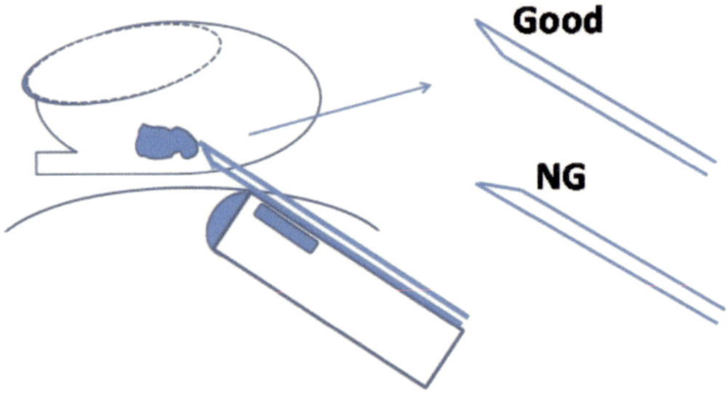

Fig. 1. Tip of needle should face on the side of rectum.

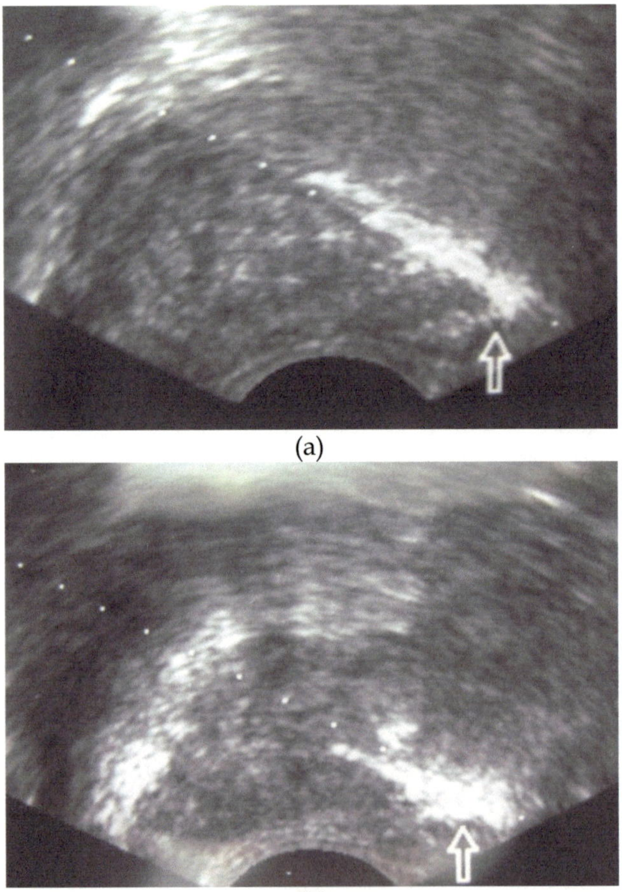

Fig. 2. A needle goes along the line of needle guide (a). And it slips away from the line when a tip of needle face on the side of prostate (b).

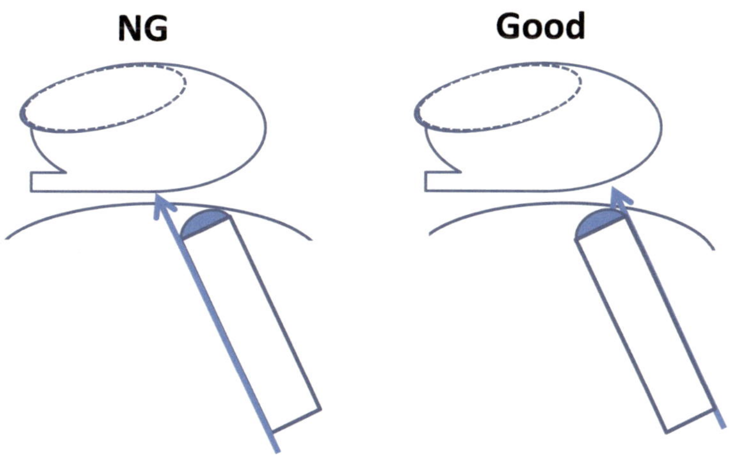

Fig. 3. On sagittal view, biopsy needle should put on the side of apex (Good).

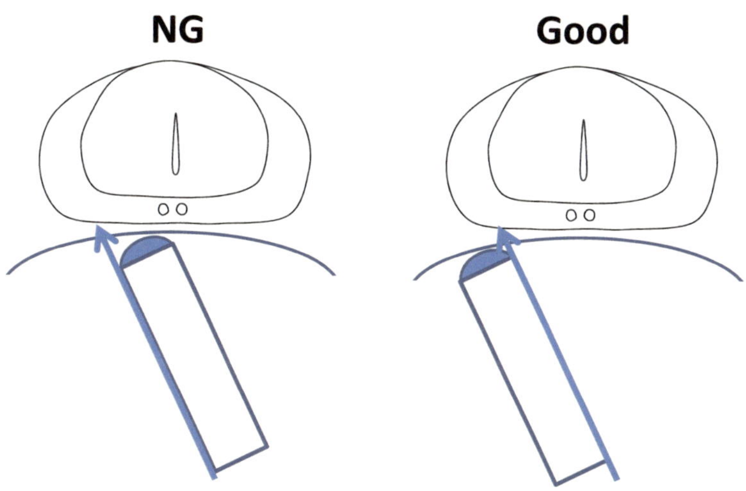

Fig. 4. On transverse view, biopsy needle should put on the right side of ultrasound probe

3. Where to fire off the needle

Biopsy itself is a relatively easy procedure. However, pathology reports sometime show the difference between experienced and unexperienced examiners. For instance, the pathology reports occasionally indicate rectal mucosa instead of prostate tissue. It happens because the beginners tend to fire off the needle before it reaches to the prostate capsule. This is the main reason for having excess rectal bleeding after biopsy. When the needle reaches to the prostate capsule, small vessels in the rectal mucosa are pushed away from the needle. The tip of the needle can easily be identified as a high echoic line on TRUS. In addition the examiner could feel the resistance at the prostate capsule (Figure 5). Immediately after the needle reaches to the prostatic capsule, it should be fired off. Even if a needle penetrates the prostatic capsule, it usually does not miss the lesion adjacent to the capsule, since the tip of the needle does not contain a cavity to collect tissue. One may try to aim at the prostatic capsule with the biopsy device to assess microscopic extraprostatic disease (Lee F, et al. 1993) but it is actually difficult to diagnose it unless extensive capsular invasion exists at the exact site of biopsy.

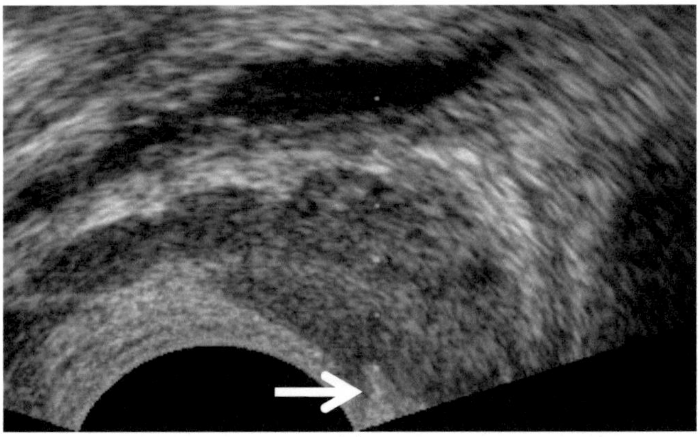

(a)

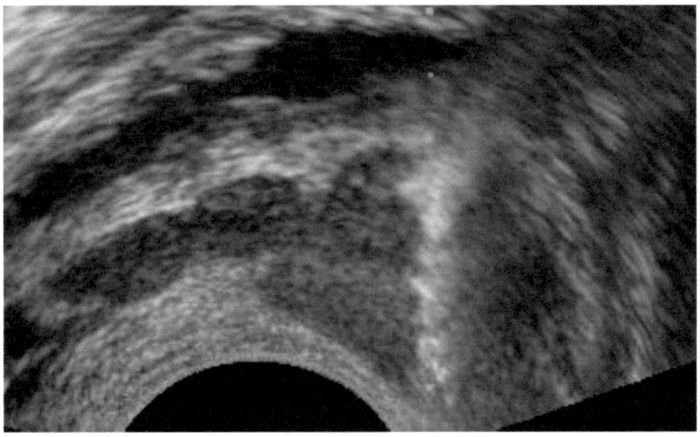

(b)

Fig. 5. A tip of needle is identified as hyperechoic line (arrow). After a tip of needle is identified at the prostatic capsule, then, it should be fired.

4. Biopsy for transition zone (TZ)

While significance of TZ biopsy is still controversial, many physicians tend to perform TZ biopsy in a setting of repeat biopsy after initial negative biopsy. Also, several investigators suggested that early prostate cancers are often located in the anterior regions at the level of apex (Figure 6). (Ishii J, et al. 2007, Takashima R, et al. 2002) Some physicians think that with using transperineal biopsy it is easy to get the appropriate samples from the TZ of the prostate. It may or may not be true. We observed many physicians performing transrectal biopsy for TZ. First, many do not insert the needle to the edge of TZ. We should insert the needle deep enough to pass the boundary between the peripheral zone and TZ, though it depends on the size of prostate gland. Because of dullness of the tip of the needle and impact of spring loaded automated biopsy gun, it looks like that a needle reaches to the inside of the TZ area. But commonly it does not reach to inside of the TZ area. The boundary between TZ and PZ can be identified by the shape of TZ, calcification and the differences of echogenecity between TZ and PZ, the locations of ejaculatory duct cysts. Because early prostate cancers tend to locate in the anterior at the level of apex, we should target more distal in the TZ as shown in Figure 7.

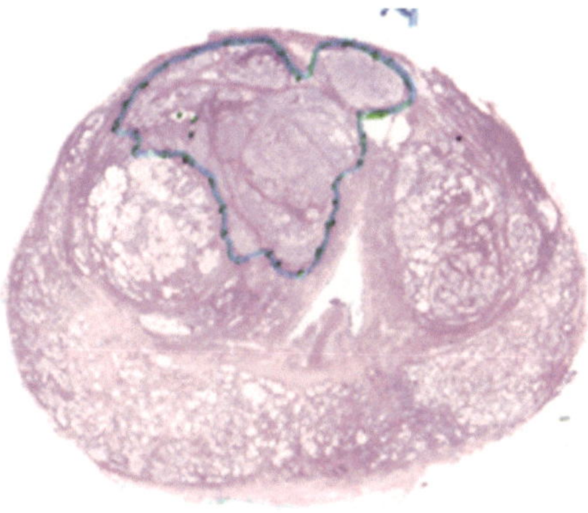

Fig. 6. Whole-mount step section of radical prostatectomy specimen shows large prostate cancer in right transition zone.

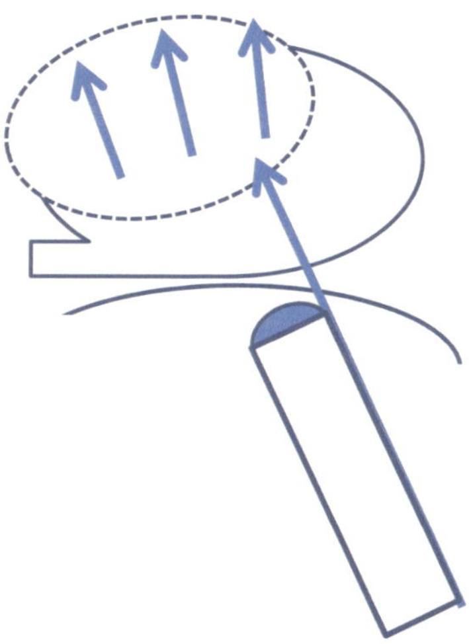

Fig. 7. A needle should be fired after it passes the boundary between TZ and PZ

5. Biopsy for far lateral prostate

Since many prostate cancers are located in the far lateral peripheral zone, it is natural to improve the detection rates of cancer when targeting this region. Therefore, for beginners it is important to identify where the "far lateral" part of the prostate is located. It is relatively easy to distinguish PZ from TZ on transverse views so that simultaneous images of both transverse and sagittal images make far lateral biopsy easy. For the sagittal images only, after identifying the center of prostate such as the line of urethra, then, slowly rotate ultrasound probe to the lateral part, so that far lateral PZ would be identified just after disappearing from TZ. For patients with middle to large prostate, far lateral PZ on sagittal images may sometimes represent only the mid-base of the prostate. To obtain biopsies from the far-lateral part of PZ at the apex, we need to slightly rotate to the center of the prostate ·

6. Biopsy for apical-apex regions

It is relatively easy to target the region of apex using the end-fire probe. However, when using the biplane probe it can sometimes be difficult because of its angle and structure of biopsy guide. Therefore, it is necessary to puncture the rectal mucosa from the distal part of the apex (Figure 8).

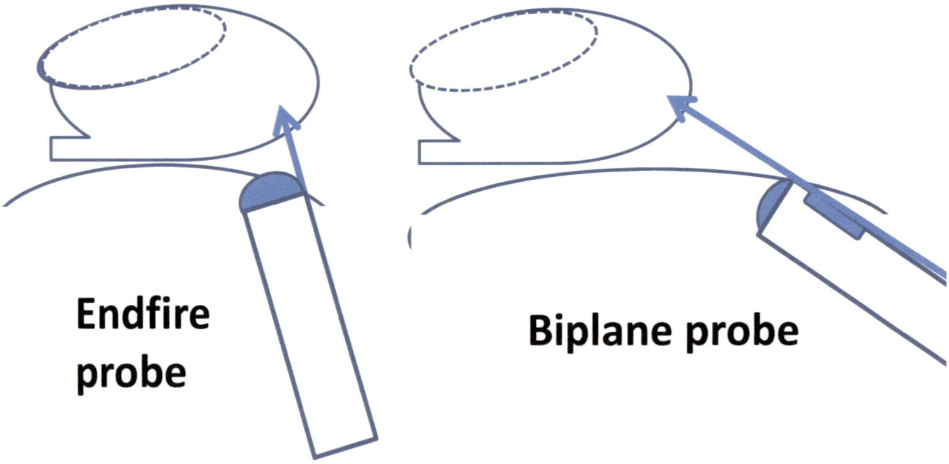

Fig. 8. It is not difficult to target the apex region with end-fire probe. With biplane probe, it may be necessary to puncture rectal mucosa distal from apex to get samples from apex.

7. Miscellaneous

Because of the length of the needle and size of device, the examiners sometime bend the needle before firing off the needle (Figure 9). This may harbor the movement of the needle, which may result in inappropriate specimens. Therefore, the examiners should avoid bending the needle and make sure to set it parallel to the biopsy device.

We sometimes observe that there are some cystic lesions in the peripheral zone which indicate the atrophic glands (Figure 10). When this region is biopsied, it is natural to get very scattered specimens.

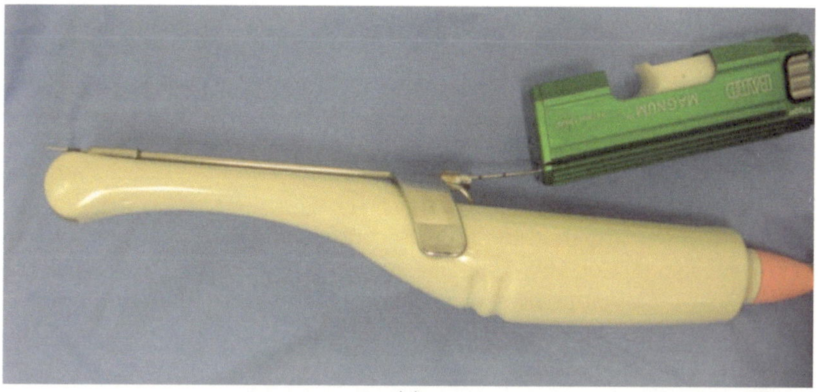

(a)

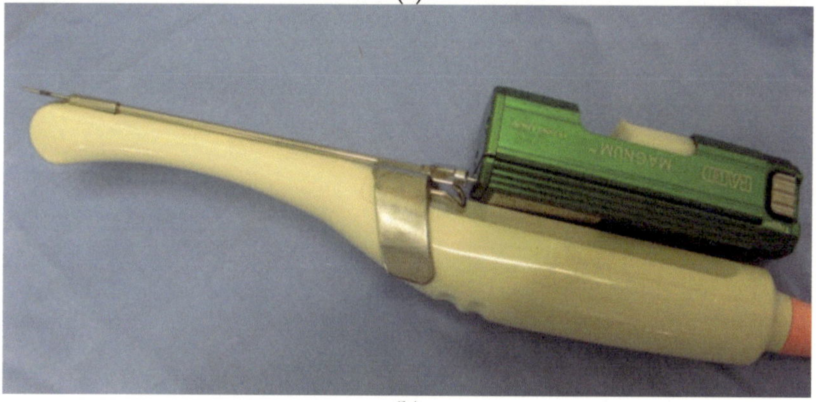

(b)

Fig. 9. When the examiners see the images during biopsy, they tend to bend a needle (a). This may result in inappropriate samples so that a needle should put parallel to the automated biopsy device(b).

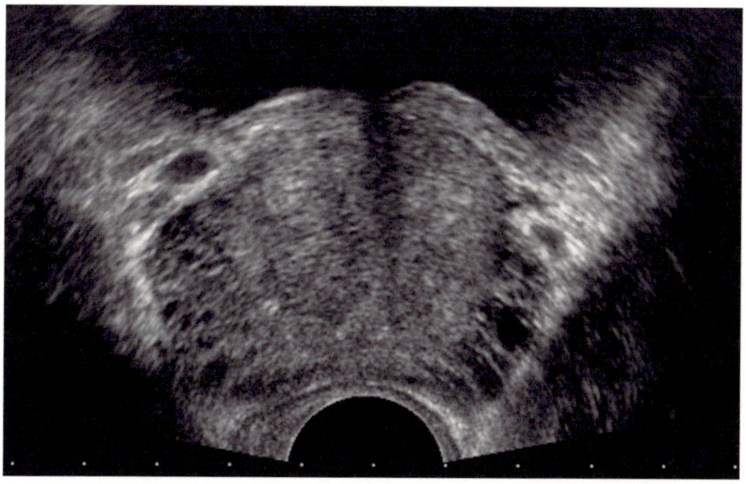

Fig. 10. Atrophic prostate glands in the peripheral zone on TRUS images.

8. References

Ishii J, et al. (2007). Significance of the craniocaudal distribution of cancer in radical prostatectomy (RP) specimens. *Int J Urol*, Vol 14, 9, pp.817-821.

Lee F, et al. (1993). The role of transrectal ultrasound-guided staging biopsy and androgen ablation therapy prior to radical prostatectomy. *Clin Invest Med* , Vol. 16, 6, pp. 458-470.

Ohori M, et al. (2003). Do impalpable (T1c) cancers visible on ultrasound differ from those not visible? *J.Urol*, Vol. 169, 3, pp.964-968.

Satake N, et al.(2010). Development and internal validation of a nomogram predicting extracapsular extension in radical prostatectomy specimens. *Int J Urol*, Vol.7, 3,pp.267-272.

Takashima R, et al. (2002). Anterior distribution of Stage T1c nonpalpable tumors in radical prostatectomy specimens. *Urology*, Vol. 59, 5, pp.692-697.

The Use of Models to Predict the Presence and Aggressiveness of Prostate Cancer on Prostate Biopsy

Stéphane Larré, Richard Bryant and Freddie Hamdy
Nuffield Department of Surgical Sciences, University of Oxford
United Kingdom

1. Introduction

Prostate cancer is the commonest male malignancy diagnosed in countries in the Western World and it represents the second commonest cause of male cancer-related death. In the United Kingdom in 2008 37,051 new cases of prostate cancer were diagnosed and this malignancy resulted in 10,168 deaths. The morbidity and mortality directly attributable to this common malignancy is considerable, however in some patients the disease is often relatively indolent. Prostate cancer is typically a disease associated with the aging male population however in some cases it may be lethal in a younger subset of men. The degree of benefit to be gained from diagnosing and treating prostate cancer is directly related to the degree of comorbidity and life expectancy of individual men. It is crucial to identify as accurately as possible men at increased risk of prostate cancer in order to improve the diagnostic performance of a prostate biopsy. Moreover it is important to be able to restrict this invasive investigation to men who are likely to benefit from treatment of this malignancy. There are currently concerns that Western clinicians and healthcare providers are over-diagnosing large numbers of men who would otherwise never have been troubled by their clinically undetectable prostate cancer. Moreover there are also concerns that large numbers of men are currently being over-treated for their prostate malignancy, resulting in treatment-related morbidity including surgical and radiotherapy complications such as erectile dysfunction and urinary incontinence. Over the last 25 years urologists and researchers have refined their skills sufficiently well to enable accurate diagnosis of a considerable proportion of prostate cancers. The contemporary challenge however is to diagnose with increased confidence those "clinically significant" cases of prostate cancer which by definition are likely to pose a threat to an individual patient if left undetected. The first part of this chapter outlines the current predictors of prostate cancer on biopsy including clinical, laboratory and research tools. Factors which may help the prediction of prostate cancer on repeat biopsy, as well as current diagnostic performance of prediction tools utilising pre- and post-biopsy data to identify men at high risk of harbouring clinically significant and aggressive prostate cancer are discussed.

2. Prediction of prostate cancer on biopsy

The current method of diagnosing prostate cancer is based upon a triad of digital rectal examination (DRE), serum prostate specific antigen (PSA) measurement, and prostate biopsy. Indications for performing a prostate biopsy include an abnormal DRE suspicious of malignancy and/or an age-specific abnormal serum PSA. At the present time the majority of cases of prostate cancer in the United Kingdom are identified following "opportunistic screening" or "case finding" whereby men present to their clinician for one of a number of other reasons and then undergo PSA-testing, ideally following appropriate and adequate counselling. A smaller proportion of cases are identified following clinical presentation with lower urinary tract symptoms or with the symptoms related to advanced prostate cancer.

There are a number of problems and controversies surrounding the diagnosis of early organ-confined prostate cancer. Firstly, the PSA test has considerable limitations in its sensitivity and specificity (Schroder et al. 2000), and the result can be difficult to interpret, particularly for non-urologists. Historically a PSA level below 4 ng/mL was considered to be "normal" however over time the upper limits of "normal" PSA were defined in an age-specific manner (table 1) (Oesterling et al. 1993).

More recently the results of the Prostate Cancer Prevention Trial (PCPT) (Thompson et al. 2003) demonstrated that there is no PSA threshold below which one can confidently exclude a diagnosis of prostate cancer. The PCPT trial protocol required "normal" men with very low levels of PSA to be biopsied at the end of the trial and it was observed that 39.2% of men with a PSA 2.1-3.0 ng/mL, 27.7% of men with a PSA 1.1-2.0 ng/mL, and 16.3% of men with a PSA <1.0 ng/mL harboured foci of adenocarcinoma of the prostate (Thompson et al. 2003). Indeed in terms of prostate cancer diagnosis and thresholds for biopsy, the PCPT trial will be remembered more for this remarkable and intriguing observation than for its observations regarding the use of finasteride for prostate cancer chemoprevention.

Age (years)	PSA ng/mL
40-49	2.5
50-59	3.5
60-69	4.5
70-79	6.5

Table 1. Age-specific upper limits of normal PSA.

Whilst some men with a PSA below the currently accepted "normal" age-specific threshold will have prostate cancer, it is also true that many men with a PSA above this threshold will not have prostate cancer as an elevated PSA can be attributable to a number of benign conditions as well apart from the presence of prostate cancer. Considerable efforts have been made to improve the sensitivity and specificity of PSA testing including the adoption of free-to-total PSA ratios, %free PSA, [-2]pro-PSA, PSA density and PSA velocity. The introduction of these parameters into prostate cancer prediction algorithms can only yield modest improvements in the diagnostic accuracy of PSA testing.

At the present time the recommendation to offer a patient a prostate biopsy in order to diagnose early organ confined disease rests with the clinician's interpretation of the PSA result and DRE findings, taking into account the patient's co-morbidity and life expectancy. The final decision to undertake a biopsy is made jointly by the patient and the clinician. This active engagement of the patient in interpreting a particular PSA result can have both benefits and negative consequences. It enables the patient to be fully engaged in this difficult decision making process. A negative consequence is the generation of a population of patients who may be described as the "worried well" i.e. men with a slightly raised PSA who have either decided not to have a biopsy or who have had negative biopsies but who still have concerns that they might harbour prostate cancer.

A number of pre-biopsy nomograms for prostate cancer risk assessment have been developed by a number of groups to predict the risk of prostate cancer on biopsy and its potential for progression. These risk calculators comprise predictive tables and nomograms and are widely available in the clinic and on the internet. They aim to aid clinicians and patients to decide whether a biopsy is indicated and also may aid treatment selection if cancer is found. The use of such nomograms requires the input of each individual patient's clinical data including parameters such as age, race, family history of prostate cancer, DRE findings, PSA level, and presence/absence of previous negative prostate biopsy (table 2).

Nomogram	Population studied	Factors included in nomogram
Cancer Risk Calculator for prostate cancer	USA	Race Age Family history of prostate cancer DRE findings PSA Previous biopsy results (if performed)
Prostate Risk Indicator	European	Risk indicator 1: Age Family history of prostate cancer Urinary symptoms Risk indicator 2: PSA Risk indicator 3: PSA TRUSS outcome DRE findings Prostate volume

Table 2. Pre-biopsy risk calculators.

The Cancer Risk Calculator for prostate cancer (Thompson et al. 2006) may be used to predict the probability of detecting prostate cancer, including those with a high Gleason Grade. This risk calculator was developed in the USA using a cohort of 5519 men in the placebo group of the PCPT who had an initial low PSA ≤3 ng/mL and had an end-of-study prostate biopsy after seven years of follow-up. This risk calculator has subsequently been adjusted to include the Prostate Cancer Antigen 3 (PCA3) score. PCA3 is a gene encoding a non-translated messenger RNA which is over-expressed in prostate cancer (Deras et al. 2008,

Marks et al. 2007). This test may be useful in evaluating men who already received one set of negative prostate biopsies.

Other adjustments include the incorporation of body mass index, the use of finasteride, percentage free PSA and [-2]pro-PSA. It should be noted that the results of the Cancer Risk Calculator for prostate cancer may not be applicable to all men as most participants in the PCPT were Caucasian, and results may not be applicable to men of other races. In addition, most men in this study underwent a sextant prostate biopsy. This has now been largely superseded by an increase in the number of systematic biopsies taken routinely (Heidenreich et al. 2010). Moreover, the risk calculator is only applicable to men aged 55 or older, without a previous history of prostate cancer and with DRE findings and PSA results less than a year old.

The Prostate Risk Indicator (www.prostatecancer-riskcalculator.com) was developed in Rotterdam and consists of 4 risk calculators, of which the first 3 predict the probability of detecting a prostate cancer (van den Bergh et al. 2008). This nomogram is based on 6288 Dutch men enrolled in the European Randomised Study of Screening for Prostate Cancer (ERSPC) (Schroder et al. 2009). The risk calculator comprises 4 risk indicators, the first 3 of which predict the possibility of a positive prostate biopsy. The first 2 prostate risk indicators produced by this group may be used by the general public whereas the other risk calculators are intended to be used by urologists during patient evaluation.

It is likely that future risk calculators developed for predicting prostate cancer risk upon performance of a prostate biopsy will incorporate the results of novel molecular diagnostic tests such as the detection of prostate cancer specific *TMPRSS2-ERG* fusion genes or *Prostate Cancer Antigen 3* (*PCA3*) in urine sediments. The *TMPRSS2-ERG* fusion gene was discovered to be specifically present in 50% of screened prostate cancer cases although there are conflicting observations regarding its association with advanced disease (Tomlins et al. 2009). A preliminary study on a limited number of patients had shown that the PCA3 test does not perform better than PSA with regards the identification of prostate cancer cases (Nyberg et al. 2010). Nevertheless, a multiplex model including TMPRSS2-ERG, PCA3, sarcosine and Annexin A3 has been shown to significantly improve diagnostic performance for this malignancy with an AUC of 0.86, whereas the AUC ranges from 0.66-0.74 for any of these markers when they are used in isolation (Cao et al. 2010). At the present time an extensive body of research is being conducted with the aim of investigating the potential clinical use of this marker and many other molecular biology tests both before and after undertaking a biopsy to diagnose prostate cancer (Shappell 2008).

Genome wide association studies (GWAS) have the capacity to detect low-risk genetic susceptibility regions associated with prostate cancer with an increased risk varying between 14-52 % (table 3) (Schumacher et al. 2011, Witte 2009). Several recent studies incorporating single nucleotide polymorphism (SNP) analyses in models predicting the diagnosis of prostate cancer upon biopsy have been published (Wiklund 2010, Aly et al. 2011, Witte 2009). Using a genetic model including 35 validated SNPs 23% of prostate biopsies could be avoided at a cost of missing a prostate cancer diagnosis in 3% of patients characterised as having an aggressive disease (Aly et al. 2011). It is hoped that in the future these approaches will reduce the number of negative prostate biopsies being performed, without reducing the detection of clinically significant prostate cancer.

Locus		Allele frequency		Association
Chr Region	SNP	Controls	Cases	Odds ratio
2p15	rs721048	0.19	0.21	1.15
2q37	rs238107965	0.25	0.29	1.14
3p12	rs2660753	0.1	0.12	1.3
6q25	rs9364554	0.29	0.33	1.21
7q21	rs6465657	0.46	0.5	1.19
8q24 (region 1)	rs1447295	0.1	0.14	1.42
8q24 (region 2)	rs16901979	0.04	0.06	1.52
8q24 (region 3)	rs6983267	0.5	0.56	1.25
10q11	rs10993994	0.38	0.46	1.38
10q26	rs4962416	0.27	0.32	1.18
11q13	rs7931342	0.51	0.56	1.21
12q13	rs902774	0.16	0.19	1.17
17q12	rs4430796	0.49	0.55	1.22
17q24	rs1859962	0.46	0.51	1.2
19q13	rs2735839	0.83	0.87	1.37
Xp11	rs5945619	0.36	0.41	1.29

Table 3. Loci associated to prostate cancer and allele frequencies

Results presented for the most significant SNPs ($p<5.10^{8}$) or those reported in multiple studies (Witte 2009, Schumacher et al. 2011).

3. Prediction of prostate cancer aggressiveness

At the time of biopsy most patients will have no clinical evidence of either lymph node involvement or distant metastasis. Patients with clinically localised disease may be offered either a radical treatment or active surveillance, and the choice depends on multiple factors reflected by D'Amico risk groups (table 4) (D'Amico et al. 1999). The assessment of the pathological stage is critical in decisions regarding appropriate treatment options. Patients more likely to have clinically insignificant or indolent prostate cancer may be good candidates for active surveillance whereas those with locally advanced disease may benefit more from a combined treatment options such as radiotherapy and androgen deprivation therapy (Mottet et al. 2011, Heidenreich et al. 2010).

The prediction of indolent prostate cancer was investigated by Kattan et al. based on criteria set by Epstein (Epstein et al. 1994) and defined as organ-confined prostate cancer less than 0.5cm3 with no Gleason grade over 4. The models were based on clinical variables (serum PSA, clinical stage and ultrasound-determined prostate volume) and others derived from the analysis of systematic biopsies of the prostate (Gleason grade, percentage of biopsy cores involved with cancer, presence of high grade cancer and total length of biopsy cores involved). Three models were developed with a c-index ranging from 64% to 79% (Kattan et al. 2003) and these validated on an external cohort resulting in a c-index ranging from 61% to 76% (Steyerberg et al. 2007). These models provide valuable information when counselling patients with prostate cancer who are considering active surveillance.

	PSA	Gleason score	Clinical stage
Low risk (all criteria present)	PSA < 10.0 ng/mL	highest biopsy Gleason score ≤6	clinical stage Tlc or T2a
Intermediate risk (any patient not at high or low risk)	PSA ≥10 but < 20 ng/mL	highest biopsy Gleason score = 7	clinical stage T2b
High risk (any criteria present)	PSA ≥ 20 ng/mL	highest biopsy Gleason score ≥ 8	clinical stage T2c/T3

Table 4. D'Amico et al risk stratification for clinically localized prostate cancer.

The local extension of prostate cancer has been investigated using multiple models. The Partin tables are the most widely used tool to predict the pathological stage of radical prostatectomy specimens based on pre-operative data (Partin et al. 1997), and have been updated many times since their creation in 1993 (Partin et al. 2001, Makarov et al. 2007) in order to correct for the effects of stage migration. The tables predict organ-confined disease, capsular penetration, seminal vesicle infiltration, and pelvic lymph node involvement using PSA level, TNM clinical stage, and Gleason score. They were modified to predict extra-capsular extension, and can assist the surgeon with decisions regarding nerve sparing during surgery (Graefen et al. 2001). This prediction tool was externally validated with a discrimination of 70% (Augustin et al. 2004), whilst the prediction of side of extra-capsular extension was accurately undertaken by Ohori et al. with a c-index ranging between 79%- to 81% (Ohori et al. 2004). Steuber et al. have also validated this prediction tool using an external population resulting in an 84% discrimination figure (Steuber et al. 2006) using the following predictors in a logistic regression model: clinical stage, pre-treatment PSA, biopsy Gleason sum score and percentage of cores positive for cancer in the biopsy specimen.

Other prognostic factors that may be predicted on prostate biopsy include the presence of seminal vesicle involvement (Koh et al. 2003, Gallina et al. 2007) with a c-index of 78% to 88% or lymph node invasion with a discrimination of 76% (Cagiannos et al. 2003, Briganti et al. 2006) Another model may be used to identify with 80% discrimination those patients at risk of lymph node invasion beyond the obturator fossa. This prediction tool may be useful indeciding whether the patients require an extended lymph node dissection (Briganti et al. 2007).

So far, Genome Wide Association Studies (GWAS) have shown little or no ability to discriminate between indolent and fatal forms of prostate cancer and this does not support their use in prediction models as reported by Aly (Aly et al. 2011). It is likely that different genetic components are involved in the initiation rather than the prognosis of prostate cancer and environmental factors may play a stronger role than genetic changes. Ongoing studies exploring the association with disease progression and prognosis rather than stage at diagnosis, will be more effective in detecting genetic risk factors for prostate cancer outcome (Wiklund 2010).

4. Evaluation of prediction tools

Prediction tools are compared using discrimination and calibration. Their use must take into consideration their clinical relevance. This can be investigated by assessing their generalisability and complexity by making adjustments for competing risks.

4.1 Discrimination

Discrimination measures the ability of a predictive tool to discriminate patients according to their outcome, for example the presence of prostate cancer versus benign pathology. Discrimination is measured using a probability score, with the lowest value being 0.5 (i.e. no better than the flip of a coin), and the highest value of 1 representing perfect discrimination (i.e. the prediction tool properly identifying the presence or absence of cancer in all patients). For binary outcomes such as the presence or absence of cancer, the discrimination value is quantified using the area under the curve (AUC). It is also assessed by the c-index for censored data (e.g. the time to biochemical recurrence after treatment) or using the Brier score (Shariat et al. 2009).

Prediction models are usually based on clinical, biological or pathological variables that impact upon the measured end point. Whilst these models are usually more accurate with the inclusion of a greater number of variables, this has to be balanced with the complexity of the model and the need to maintain clinical relevance. The risk of occurrence of the event of interest may change over time. For example the risk of observing biochemical progression at any time after treatment is highest just after treatment, and decreases with the disease free interval. Prediction models therefore need to take these factors into account to ensure accuracy.

4.2 Calibration

Whereas discrimination is an overall measurement of prediction tool accuracy, the term calibration reflects the precision of the test at an individual level. It compares the predicted results for each patient with the observed values. In the case of prostate cancer this may be used to predict the presence of a biochemical recurrence. Calibration is represented using two curves, one being the ideal curve (45 degree slope line) and the other representing the observed test result (figure 1). In an ideal model both curves will overlap. It is useful to identify graphically whether the model is well calibrated for all events or only for some events. It may be accurate for short term prediction of biochemical recurrence, but not for long term prediction of disease outcome (Figure 1). Calibration is usually good when applied to the population used to create the prediction model, but not necessarily to another population in which the clinical variables may differ. It is therefore important that the model is validated on an external population. If the discrimination and calibration are similar it is more likely that the predicting model is robust and therefore generalizable (Shariat et al. 2009).

The blue line represents the result of an ideal prediction model. The red line represents time to biochemical recurrence observed compared with time to biochemical recurrence predicted. Time to recurrence was overestimated at 5 years, and underestimated at 10 years. The curve also shows that the model is more accurate in predicting early than late recurrence.

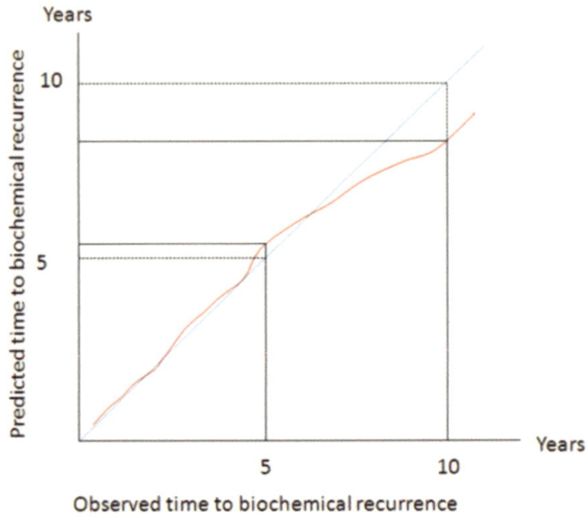

Fig. 1. Example of calibration curve.

4.3 Clinical relevance
4.3.1 Generalizability
The clinical relevance of a prediction tool depends not only on its intrinsic discrimination and calibration performance but also on its generalizability, level of complexity and adjustment for competing risks. It is worth noting that any result applies to the population analysed, and extrapolation to another population should be used with caution. Where a model is more complex and integrates more clinical variables, it is more likely to be generalizable since the model usually adjusts the results according to these variables. Before using a prediction tool prospectively, it is recommended to test the performance of the model on retrospective cohorts. When this approach was applied to populations of patient undergoing radical prostatectomy using the Kattan nomogram (Kattan et al. 1998) the discrimination varied between 0.67-0.83 (Roupret et al. 2009) indicating a poor generalizability. Reduced generalizability may be observed when the stages of cancer at diagnosis are different between populations.

The performance of a predictive tool based on a screened population may differ when used on a non-screened population because the stage at diagnosis tends to be higher in the latter group of patients (Steyerberg et al. 2007). Another common cause of reduced generalizability is the use of models based on a historical cohort of patients treated many years previously. Patient characteristics at diagnosis may have changed over time and new treatments may have impacted on the target point risk. Once again the validation of recent cohorts is necessary unless the prediction model has been modified to take into account the differences observed in more recent cohorts (Greene et al. 2004, Shariat et al. 2009).

4.3.2 Level of complexity
Another parameter impacting on the clinical relevance of prediction tools is the complexity of the model used. Some models are accurate but may require complex algorithms and include large numbers of variables. The use of the model will therefore require computer support and all variables need to be entered manually, which may be time consuming. Some

variables, such as biomarker information, may not be routinely available and the model may not be useful in daily clinical practice. One example is the use of PSA kinetics such as PSA velocity or doubling time which require several measurements, and PSA density, requiring prostate volume information which may not be available routinely (Shariat et al. 2009).

4.3.3 Adjustment for competing risks

Predicting the risk of prostate cancer progression may be irrelevant in the presence of substantial competing comorbidties which could lead to non cancer-specific mortality prior to any progression event. It is therefore of paramount importance to account for competing risks in any predictive model. Adjustment is important when there is a particular risk of over-treatment where intervention can be associated with significant morbidity. (Nielsen et al. 2007).

4.4 Comparison of existing prediction models

When new prediction models are developed they should be compared with existing tools and validated before they are introduced to routine clinical practice. New prediction tests need to be compared to the best current prediction tools using similar populations. These comparisons are best made by assessing discrimination and calibration as highlighted earlier in this chapter, to offer an unbiased and objective assessment of the new model and it is clinical utility. This systematic head-to-head comparison of prediction tools is considered a better approach than a simple comparison of the concordance index or the AUC, although the results may be different depending on the methods used for comparison (Lughezzani et al. 2010).

Comparisons of prediction tests should ideally include a decision analysis to assess the impact of the prediction tool in clinical practice. One of the most simple and efficient methods is a decision curve analysis described previously (Vickers 2008). This method takes into consideration the probability of false positives or false negatives. For example, when considering the prediction of prostate cancer based on a model, a false positive result describes a patient wrongly assigned to have prostate cancer with a negative biopsy result. Conversely a false negative result describes a patient wrongly assigned to not having cancer, who will be denied a prostate biopsy. These false results are given a harm score, with for instance a false negative result for a prostate biopsy with subsequent deleterious delayed treatment. This latter situation is considered four-fold more harmful than a false positive outcome resulting in an unnecessary prostate biopsy. Clinical consequences of the different models can therefore also be compared in terms of the potential harm they may cause. Such analysis is best performed during the late stages of model development before the tool is implemented clinically (Lughezzani et al. 2010).

4.5 Prediction tools of the future

Many of the current prostate cancer prediction tools are imperfect, lack discrimination and are often difficult to use in daily clinical practice. The addition of other potentially informative clinical and pathological data has not resulted in significant improvement of current models. Nevertheless further improvement of existing models is potentially possible by implementing imaging data, use of biomarkers, and the use of "smart" electronic medical records.

Non-invasive imaging in the field of prostate cancer diagnosis, staging and treatment planning has gained widespread acceptance in recent years. Magnetic resonance imaging (MRI) data has been implemented in several prediction tools in order to accurately identify organ-confined prostate cancer (Wang et al. 2007) or to detect clinically relevant disease (Shukla-Dave et al. 2007), however to date this has not been properly investigated in the diagnosis of prostate cancer before biopsy.

Over the past few years numerous reports identified promising new biomarkers associated with the presence of prostate cancer which correlate with its aggressive behaviour (Reed and Parekh 2010, Shappell 2008). The introduction of urine and blood biomarkers in predictions tools was investigated to predict more accurately disease relapse after radical prostatectomy (Shariat et al. 2008a, Shariat et al. 2008b). Clinical practice is currently based on the interpretation of a handful of parameters by physicians without automated support, but it has been demonstrated that prediction models may perform better than the clinician regardless of their levels of expertise (Ross et al. 2002, Walz et al. 2007). Improvements in technology now make it possible to assess rapidly large amounts of molecular biology data at a greatly reduced cost compared to the recent past. The use of computational algorithms to analyse the results of biomarker tests, and the use of evidence-based data to support this approach, is likely to improve patient care but this has not yet been confirmed.

In the future, these algorithms may be incorporated into "smart" electronic medical records with the ability to analyse a patient's individual risk of harbouring clinically significant disease, using new and conventional clinico-pathological data such as pathology results which will need to be reported as specific fields (e.g. primary and secondary Gleason scores) as well as in the conventional manner as a text result. This approach requires modifications of clinical practice with the wide implementation of electronic medical records. Algorithms could then be refined by merging data from multiple centres with different patient populations, and the integration of other investigations such as multiparametric MRI scanning.

5. Conclusion

Currently, many parameters can be used to estimate an individual's risk of harbouring prostate cancer on biopsy. Pre- and post-biopsy factors require further investigation to determine whether the cancer detected is potentially aggressive. This is critical to predict whether a prostate biopsy is likely to offer real benefit to individual patients, and to guide therapeutic options. Despite the multiple limitations described above, predictive tools could, in the future provide personalised and evidenced based information, including molecular tumour profiling of individual patients to improve the outcome of such a common and ubiquitous disease as prostate cancer.

6. References

Aly, M., F. Wiklund, J. Xu, W. B. Isaacs, M. Eklund, M. D'Amato, J. Adolfsson & H. Gronberg (2011) Polygenic Risk Score Improves Prostate Cancer Risk Prediction: Results from the Stockholm-1 Cohort Study. *Eur Urol,* Vol., No. 2011/02/08, pp.

Augustin, H., T. Eggert, S. Wenske, P. I. Karakiewicz, J. Palisaar, F. Daghofer, H. Huland & M. Graefen (2004) Comparison of accuracy between the Partin tables of 1997 and 2001 to predict final pathological stage in clinically localized prostate cancer. *J Urol,* Vol. 171, No. 1, 2003/12/11, pp. 177-81.

Briganti, A., F. K. Chun, A. Salonia, G. Zanni, A. Gallina, F. Deho, N. Suardi, L. F. Da Pozzo, L. Valiquette, P. Rigatti, F. Montorsi & P. I. Karakiewicz (2007) A nomogram for staging of exclusive nonobturator lymph node metastases in men with localized prostate cancer. *Eur Urol,* Vol. 51, No. 1, pp. 112-9; discussion 119-20.

Briganti, A., F. K. Chun, A. Salonia, G. Zanni, V. Scattoni, L. Valiquette, P. Rigatti, F. Montorsi & P. I. Karakiewicz (2006) Validation of a nomogram predicting the probability of lymph node invasion among patients undergoing radical prostatectomy and an extended pelvic lymphadenectomy. *Eur Urol,* Vol. 49, No. 6, 2006/03/15, pp. 1019-26; discussion 1026-7.

Cagiannos, I., P. Karakiewicz, J. A. Eastham, M. Ohori, F. Rabbani, C. Gerigk, V. Reuter, M. Graefen, P. G. Hammerer, A. Erbersdobler, H. Huland, P. Kupelian, E. Klein, D. I. Quinn, S. M. Henshall, J. J. Grygiel, R. L. Sutherland, P. D. Stricker, C. G. Morash, P. T. Scardino & M. W. Kattan (2003) A preoperative nomogram identifying decreased risk of positive pelvic lymph nodes in patients with prostate cancer. *J Urol,* Vol. 170, No. 5, pp. 1798-803.

Cancer_Research_UK (2011) Latest UK Cancer Incidence (2008) and Mortality (2008) Summary. *http://info.cancerresearchuk.org/prod_consump/groups/cr_common/@nre/@sta/documents/generalcontent/cr_074228.pdf*

Cao, D. L., D. W. Ye, H. L. Zhang, Y. Zhu, Y. X. Wang & X. D. Yao (2010) A multiplex model of combining gene-based, protein-based, and metabolite-based with positive and negative markers in urine for the early diagnosis of prostate cancer. *Prostate,* Vol., No. 2010/10/20, pp.

D'Amico, A. V., R. Whittington, S. B. Malkowicz, J. Fondurulia, M. H. Chen, I. Kaplan, C. J. Beard, J. E. Tomaszewski, A. A. Renshaw, A. Wein & C. N. Coleman (1999) Pretreatment nomogram for prostate-specific antigen recurrence after radical prostatectomy or external-beam radiation therapy for clinically localized prostate cancer. *J Clin Oncol,* Vol. 17, No. 1, pp. 168-72.

Deras, I. L., S. M. Aubin, A. Blase, J. R. Day, S. Koo, A. W. Partin, W. J. Ellis, L. S. Marks, Y. Fradet, H. Rittenhouse & J. Groskopf (2008) PCA3: a molecular urine assay for predicting prostate biopsy outcome. *J Urol,* Vol. 179, No. 4, 2008/02/26, pp. 1587-92.

Epstein, J. I., M. J. Carmichael, A. W. Partin & P. C. Walsh (1994) Small high grade adenocarcinoma of the prostate in radical prostatectomy specimens performed for nonpalpable disease: pathogenetic and clinical implications. *J Urol,* Vol. 151, No. 6, pp. 1587-92.

Gallina, A., F. K. Chun, A. Briganti, S. F. Shariat, F. Montorsi, A. Salonia, A. Erbersdobler, P. Rigatti, L. Valiquette, H. Huland, M. Graefen & P. I. Karakiewicz (2007) Development and split-sample validation of a nomogram predicting the probability of seminal vesicle invasion at radical prostatectomy. *Eur Urol,* Vol. 52, No. 1, pp. 98-105.

Graefen, M., A. Haese, U. Pichlmeier, P. G. Hammerer, J. Noldus, K. Butz, A. Erbersdobler, R. P. Henke, U. Michl, S. Fernandez & H. Huland (2001) A validated strategy for side specific prediction of organ confined prostate cancer: a tool to select for nerve sparing radical prostatectomy. *J Urol,* Vol. 165, No. 3, pp. 857-63.

Greene, K. L., M. V. Meng, E. P. Elkin, M. R. Cooperberg, D. J. Pasta, M. W. Kattan, K. Wallace & P. R. Carroll (2004) Validation of the Kattan preoperative nomogram for prostate cancer recurrence using a community based cohort: results from cancer of the prostate strategic urological research endeavor (capsure). *J Urol,* Vol. 171, No. 6 Pt 1, pp. 2255-9.

Heidenreich, A., J. Bellmunt, M. Bolla, S. Joniau, M. Mason, V. Matveev, N. Mottet, H. P. Schmid, T. van der Kwast, T. Wiegel & F. Zattoni (2010) EAU Guidelines on Prostate Cancer. Part 1: Screening, Diagnosis, and Treatment of Clinically Localised Disease. *Eur Urol,* Vol., No. 2010/11/09, pp.

Kattan, M. W., J. A. Eastham, A. M. Stapleton, T. M. Wheeler & P. T. Scardino (1998) A preoperative nomogram for disease recurrence following radical prostatectomy for prostate cancer. *J Natl Cancer Inst,* Vol. 90, No. 10, pp. 766-71.

Kattan, M. W., J. A. Eastham, T. M. Wheeler, N. Maru, P. T. Scardino, A. Erbersdobler, M. Graefen, H. Huland, H. Koh, S. F. Shariat, K. M. Slawin & M. Ohori (2003) Counseling men with prostate cancer: a nomogram for predicting the presence of small, moderately differentiated, confined tumors. *J Urol,* Vol. 170, No. 5, pp. 1792-7.

Koh, H., M. W. Kattan, P. T. Scardino, K. Suyama, N. Maru, K. Slawin, T. M. Wheeler & M. Ohori (2003) A nomogram to predict seminal vesicle invasion by the extent and location of cancer in systematic biopsy results. *J Urol,* Vol. 170, No. 4 Pt 1, pp. 1203-8.

Lughezzani, G., L. Budaus, H. Isbarn, M. Sun, P. Perrotte, A. Haese, F. K. Chun, T. Schlomm, T. Steuber, H. Heinzer, H. Huland, F. Montorsi, M. Graefen & P. I. Karakiewicz (2010) Head-to-head comparison of the three most commonly used preoperative models for prediction of biochemical recurrence after radical prostatectomy. *Eur Urol,* Vol. 57, No. 4, 2009/12/19, pp. 562-8.

Makarov, D. V., B. J. Trock, E. B. Humphreys, L. A. Mangold, P. C. Walsh, J. I. Epstein & A. W. Partin (2007) Updated nomogram to predict pathologic stage of prostate cancer given prostate-specific antigen level, clinical stage, and biopsy Gleason score (Partin tables) based on cases from 2000 to 2005. *Urology,* Vol. 69, No. 6, pp. 1095-101.

Marks, L. S., Y. Fradet, I. L. Deras, A. Blase, J. Mathis, S. M. Aubin, A. T. Cancio, M. Desaulniers, W. J. Ellis, H. Rittenhouse & J. Groskopf (2007) PCA3 molecular urine assay for prostate cancer in men undergoing repeat biopsy. *Urology,* Vol. 69, No. 3, pp. 532-5.

Mottet, N., J. Bellmunt, M. Bolla, S. Joniau, M. Mason, V. Matveev, H. P. Schmid, T. Van der Kwast, T. Wiegel, F. Zattoni & A. Heidenreich (2011) EAU Guidelines on Prostate Cancer. Part II: Treatment of Advanced, Relapsing, and Castration-Resistant Prostate Cancer. *Eur Urol,* Vol., No. 2011/02/15, pp.

Nielsen, M. E., S. F. Shariat, P. I. Karakiewicz, Y. Lotan, C. G. Rogers, G. E. Amiel, P. J. Bastian, A. Vazina, A. Gupta, S. P. Lerner, A. I. Sagalowsky, M. P. Schoenberg & G. S. Palapattu (2007) Advanced age is associated with poorer bladder cancer-specific survival in patients treated with radical cystectomy. *Eur Urol,* Vol. 51, No. 3, 2006/11/23, pp. 699-706; discussion 706-8.

Nyberg, M., D. Ulmert, A. Lindgren, U. Lindstrom, P. A. Abrahamsson & A. Bjartell (2010) PCA3 as a diagnostic marker for prostate cancer: a validation study on a Swedish patient population. *Scand J Urol Nephrol,* Vol. 44, No. 6, 2010/10/22, pp. 378-83.

Oesterling, J. E., W. H. Cooner, S. J. Jacobsen, H. A. Guess & M. M. Lieber (1993) Influence of patient age on the serum PSA concentration. An important clinical observation. *Urol Clin North Am,* Vol. 20, No. 4, pp. 671-80.

Ohori, M., M. W. Kattan, H. Koh, N. Maru, K. M. Slawin, S. Shariat, M. Muramoto, V. E. Reuter, T. M. Wheeler & P. T. Scardino (2004) Predicting the presence and side of extracapsular extension: a nomogram for staging prostate cancer. *J Urol,* Vol. 171, No. 5, pp. 1844-9; discussion 1849.

Partin, A. W., M. W. Kattan, E. N. Subong, P. C. Walsh, K. J. Wojno, J. E. Oesterling, P. T. Scardino & J. D. Pearson (1997) Combination of prostate-specific antigen, clinical stage, and Gleason score to predict pathological stage of localized prostate cancer. A multi-institutional update. *Jama,* Vol. 277, No. 18, pp. 1445-51.

Partin, A. W., L. A. Mangold, D. M. Lamm, P. C. Walsh, J. I. Epstein & J. D. Pearson (2001) Contemporary update of prostate cancer staging nomograms (Partin Tables) for the new millennium. *Urology,* Vol. 58, No. 6, pp. 843-8.

Reed, A. B. & D. J. Parekh (2010) Biomarkers for prostate cancer detection. *Expert Rev Anticancer Ther,* Vol. 10, No. 1, 2009/12/18, pp. 103-14.

Ross, P. L., C. Gerigk, M. Gonen, O. Yossepowitch, I. Cagiannos, P. C. Sogani, P. T. Scardino & M. W. Kattan (2002) Comparisons of nomograms and urologists' predictions in prostate cancer. *Semin Urol Oncol,* Vol. 20, No. 2, 2002/05/16, pp. 82-8.

Roupret, M., V. Hupertan, E. Comperat, S. J. Drouin, V. Phe, E. Xylinas, D. Demanse, M. Sibony, F. Richard & O. Cussenot (2009) Cross-cultural validation of a prognostic tool: example of the Kattan preoperative nomogram as a predictor of prostate cancer recurrence after radical prostatectomy. *BJU Int,* Vol. 104, No. 6, 2009/03/04, pp. 813-7; discussion 817-8.

Schroder, F. H., J. Hugosson, M. J. Roobol, T. L. Tammela, S. Ciatto, V. Nelen, M. Kwiatkowski, M. Lujan, H. Lilja, M. Zappa, L. J. Denis, F. Recker, A. Berenguer, L. Maattanen, C. H. Bangma, G. Aus, A. Villers, X. Rebillard, T. van der Kwast, B. G. Blijenberg, S. M. Moss, H. J. de Koning & A. Auvinen (2009) Screening and prostate-cancer mortality in a randomized European study. *N Engl J Med,* Vol. 360, No. 13, 2009/03/20, pp. 1320-8.

Schroder, F. H., I. van der Cruijsen-Koeter, H. J. de Koning, A. N. Vis, R. F. Hoedemaeker & R. Kranse (2000) Prostate cancer detection at low prostate specific antigen. *J Urol,* Vol. 163, No. 3, pp. 806-12.

Schumacher, F. R., S. I. Berndt, A. Siddiq, K. B. Jacobs, Z. Wang, S. Lindstrom, V. L. Stevens, C. Chen, A. M. Mondul, R. C. Travis, D. O. Stram, R. A. Eeles, D. F. Easton, G. Giles, J. L. Hopper, D. E. Neal, F. C. Hamdy, J. L. Donovan, K. Muir, A. Amin Al Olama, Z. Kote-Jarai, M. Guy, G. Severi, H. Gronberg, W. B. Isaacs, R. Karlsson, F. Wiklund, J. Xu, N. E. Allen, G. L. Andriole, A. Barricarte, H. Boeing, H. B. Bueno-de-Mesquita, E. D. Crawford, W. R. Diver, C. A. Gonzalez, J. M. Gaziano, E. L. Giovannucci, M. Johansson, L. Le Marchand, J. Ma, S. Sieri, P. Stattin, M. J. Stampfer, A. Tjonneland, P. Vineis, J. Virtamo, U. Vogel, S. J. Weinstein, M. Yeager, M. J. Thun, L. N. Kolonel, B. E. Henderson, D. Albanes, R. B. Hayes, H. S. Feigelson, E. Riboli, D. J. Hunter, S. J. Chanock, C. A. Haiman & P. Kraft (2011) Genome-wide association study identifies new prostate cancer susceptibility loci. *Hum Mol Genet,* Vol., No. 2011/07/12, pp.

Shappell, S. B. (2008) Clinical utility of prostate carcinoma molecular diagnostic tests. *Rev Urol,* Vol. 10, No. 1, 2008/05/13, pp. 44-69.

Shariat, S. F., J. A. Karam, J. Walz, C. G. Roehrborn, F. Montorsi, V. Margulis, F. Saad, K. M. Slawin & P. I. Karakiewicz (2008a) Improved prediction of disease relapse after radical prostatectomy through a panel of preoperative blood-based biomarkers. *Clin Cancer Res,* Vol. 14, No. 12, 2008/06/19, pp. 3785-91.

Shariat, S. F., M. W. Kattan, A. J. Vickers, P. I. Karakiewicz & P. T. Scardino (2009) Critical review of prostate cancer predictive tools. *Future Oncol,* Vol. 5, No. 10, 2009/12/17, pp. 1555-84.

Shariat, S. F., J. Walz, C. G. Roehrborn, A. R. Zlotta, P. Perrotte, N. Suardi, F. Saad & P. I. Karakiewicz (2008b) External validation of a biomarker-based preoperative nomogram predicts biochemical recurrence after radical prostatectomy. *J Clin Oncol,* Vol. 26, No. 9, 2008/03/20, pp. 1526-31.

Shukla-Dave, A., H. Hricak, M. W. Kattan, D. Pucar, K. Kuroiwa, H. N. Chen, J. Spector, J. A. Koutcher, K. L. Zakian & P. T. Scardino (2007) The utility of magnetic resonance imaging and spectroscopy for predicting insignificant prostate cancer: an initial analysis. *BJU Int,* Vol. 99, No. 4, 2007/01/17, pp. 786-93.

Stanford, J. L., L. M. FitzGerald, S. K. McDonnell, E. E. Carlson, L. M. McIntosh, K. Deutsch, L. Hood, E. A. Ostrander & D. J. Schaid (2009) Dense genome-wide SNP linkage scan in 301 hereditary prostate cancer families identifies multiple regions with suggestive evidence for linkage. *Hum Mol Genet,* Vol. 18, No. 10, 2009/03/03, pp. 1839-48.

Steuber, T., M. Graefen, A. Haese, A. Erbersdobler, F. K. Chun, T. Schlom, P. Perrotte, H. Huland & P. I. Karakiewicz (2006) Validation of a nomogram for prediction of side specific extracapsular extension at radical prostatectomy. *J Urol,* Vol. 175, No. 3 Pt 1, 2006/02/14, pp. 939-44; discussion 944.

Steyerberg, E. W., M. J. Roobol, M. W. Kattan, T. H. van der Kwast, H. J. de Koning & F. H. Schroder (2007) Prediction of indolent prostate cancer: validation and updating of a prognostic nomogram. *J Urol,* Vol. 177, No. 1, pp. 107-12; discussion 112.

Thompson, I. M., D. P. Ankerst, C. Chi, P. J. Goodman, C. M. Tangen, M. S. Lucia, Z. Feng, H. L. Parnes & C. A. Coltman, Jr. (2006) Assessing prostate cancer risk: results from the Prostate Cancer Prevention Trial. *J Natl Cancer Inst,* Vol. 98, No. 8, 2006/04/20, pp. 529-34.

Thompson, I. M., P. J. Goodman, C. M. Tangen, M. S. Lucia, G. J. Miller, L. G. Ford, M. M. Lieber, R. D. Cespedes, J. N. Atkins, S. M. Lippman, S. M. Carlin, A. Ryan, C. M. Szczepanek, J. J. Crowley & C. A. Coltman, Jr. (2003) The influence of finasteride on the development of prostate cancer. *N Engl J Med,* Vol. 349, No. 3, pp. 215-24.

Tomlins, S. A., A. Bjartell, A. M. Chinnaiyan, G. Jenster, R. K. Nam, M. A. Rubin & J. A. Schalken (2009) ETS gene fusions in prostate cancer: from discovery to daily clinical practice. *Eur Urol,* Vol. 56, No. 2, 2009/05/05, pp. 275-86.

van den Bergh, R. C., M. J. Roobol, T. Wolters, P. J. van Leeuwen & F. H. Schroder (2008) The Prostate Cancer Prevention Trial and European Randomized Study of Screening for Prostate Cancer risk calculators indicating a positive prostate biopsy: a comparison. *BJU Int,* Vol. 102, No. 9, 2008/08/22, pp. 1068-73.

Vickers, A. J. (2008) Decision analysis for the evaluation of diagnostic tests, prediction models and molecular markers. *Am Stat,* Vol. 62, No. 4, 2009/01/10, pp. 314-320.

Walz, J., A. Gallina, P. Perrotte, C. Jeldres, Q. D. Trinh, G. C. Hutterer, M. Traumann, A. Ramirez, S. F. Shariat, M. McCormack, J. P. Perreault, F. Benard, L. Valiquette, F. Saad & P. I. Karakiewicz (2007) Clinicians are poor raters of life-expectancy before radical prostatectomy or definitive radiotherapy for localized prostate cancer. *BJU Int,* Vol. 100, No. 6, pp. 1254-8.

Wang, L., H. Hricak, M. W. Kattan, H. N. Chen, K. Kuroiwa, H. F. Eisenberg & P. T. Scardino (2007) Prediction of seminal vesicle invasion in prostate cancer: incremental value of adding endorectal MR imaging to the Kattan nomogram. *Radiology,* Vol. 242, No. 1, pp. 182-8.

Wiklund, F. (2010) Prostate cancer genomics: can we distinguish between indolent and fatal disease using genetic markers? *Genome Med,* Vol. 2, No. 7, 2010/07/30, pp. 45.

Witte, J. S. (2009) Prostate cancer genomics: towards a new understanding. *Nat Rev Genet,* Vol. 10, No. 2, 2008/12/24, pp. 77-82.

6

The Role of Anticoagulant Therapy During Prostate Biopsy

F. Zaman, C. Bach, P. Kumar, I. Junaid,
N. Buchholz and J. Masood
Barts and the London NHS Trust
UK

1. Introduction

Since the advent of PSA (prostate specific antigen) in the early 1980s there has been a dramatic increase in the diagnosis of prostate cancer and transrectal ultrasound-guided biopsy (TRUS) has emerged as one of the most frequently performed urological procedures. The most common complications are haemorrhagic. Haematuria (12.5 to 80%), haematospermia (5.1 to 89%), and rectal bleeding (1.3 to 58.6%) have been reported to occur [1-3]. However, these bleeding symptoms generally resolve without treatment. Factors other than biopsy can influence the bleeding complication rate like anticoagulant medication and some medical conditions.

Older patients constitute the main target group for prostate cancer screening and subsequently undergo prostate biopsy. At the same time cardiovascular disease most commonly affects the elderly who require low dose acetylsalicylic acid (ASA, 75 mg, once daily), clopidogrel or warfarin as the mainstay of primary and secondary prophylaxis for coronary and peripheral vascular disease. The optimal management of patients who receive low doses (up to 100 mg) of acetylsalicylic acid (ASA) / clopidogrel / warfarin and who are scheduled to undergo prostatic biopsy is still controversial. The approaches being implemented in every day clinical practice vary and include discontinuation of anticoagulation therapy, replacement with low-molecular weight heparin and continuing ASA during peri-procedural period.

Little evidence is available and standardized comprehensive guidelines have not been developed to determine how to manage antiplatelet therapy or warfarin in surgical patients.

2. Literature review

To our knowledge there has not been a comprehensive review of this topic for evaluating haemostatic status before interventions. Here we shall provide a summation of literature regarding the patients coagulation status, detail patient conditions that can affect coagulation, and review common medications used to modify the haemostatic system to prevent complications.

2.1 Antiplatelet medication – ASA (acetylsalicylic acid, aspirin)

The mechanism of aspirin's antiplatelet action was first described in 1971 by the British pharmacologist John Vane. It inhibits the enzyme cyclooxygenase (COX), thereby preventing the production of prostaglandins. Subsequently, researchers identified two COX isoenzymes, COX-1, and COX-2. Cyclooxygenase is required for prostaglandin and thromboxane synthesis. Prostaglandins produced by COX-2 primarily trigger pain and inflammation, while those produced by COX-1 perform maintenance functions such as promoting normal platelet activity.

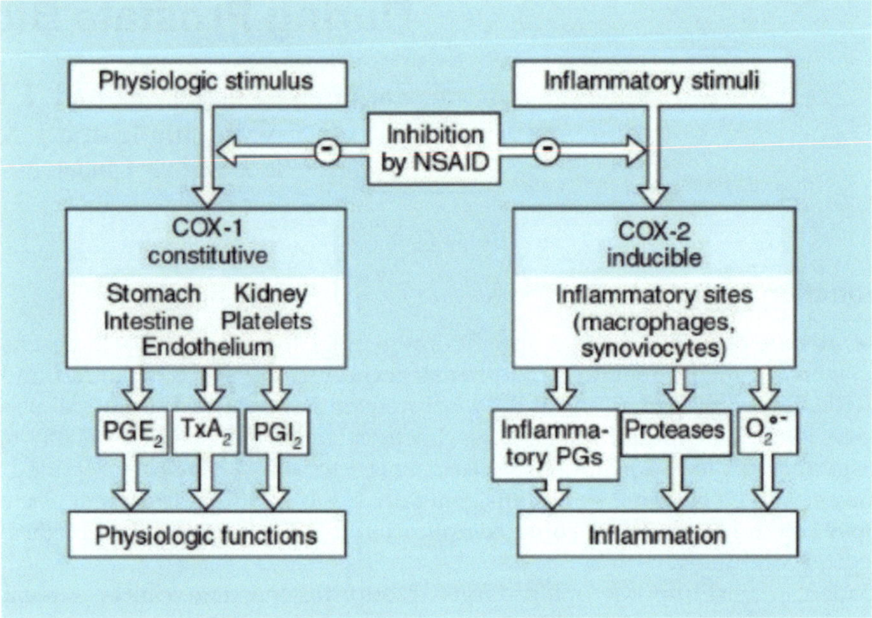

Fig. 1. Showing action of COX-1 and COX-2 enzyme - the products of COX-1 tend to have so-called housekeeping functions. This enzyme is constitutively present in cells. In contrast, the COX-2 enzyme is induced in cells in response to inflammatory stimuli. The products of both enzymes tend to cause inflammation.

In platelets, the COX-1 enzyme produces thromboxane A_2, which causes platelets to aggregate. Aspirin acts as an acetylating agent where an acetyl group is covalently attached to a serine residue in the active site of the COX enzyme. Aspirin, by inhibiting the COX-1 enzyme and therefore the production of thromboxane A_2, derives a potential antiplatelet effect which lasts for the life of the platelet (7-10 days). Because platelets do not have a nucleus and therefore contain no DNA, no new cyclo-oxygenase can be produced, so the effect of aspirin on platelets persists until enough new platelets have been formed to replace affected ones. This takes approximately seven to ten days, i.e. the lifespan of a platelet as we mentioned earlier. Therefore, the risk of increased bleeding, caused by aspirin, persists for some days after aspirin treatment has been stopped. COX-1 catalyzes the synthesis of thromboxane A_2 (Tx-A_2), which causes platelet activation, vasoconstriction, and smooth muscle proliferation. Tx-A_2 levels are elevated in conditions associated with platelet activation, including unstable angina and cerebral ischemia. Conversely, COX-2 controls the synthesis of prostacyclin (PGI_2), a local platelet regulator with an effect opposite to that of Tx-A_2. PGI_2 is produced as a compensatory response to increases in Tx-A_2 during ischemic events.

Aspirin at low doses selectively inhibits the formation of Tx-A_2 without inhibiting the basal biosynthesis of cardioprotective PGI_2. This effect is irreversible because platelets are enucleate and, thus, unable to resynthesize COX-1. This makes aspirin different from other NSAIDs (such as diclofenac and ibuprofen), which are reversible.

2.1.1 Mechanism of action of aspirin (C9H8O4)

Aspirin is rapidly absorbed in the stomach and upper small intestine, primarily by passive diffusion of nondissociated acetylsalicylic acid across gastrointestinal membranes. It takes 30-40 minutes to reach plasma peak level for an uncoated aspirin whereas three to four hours for enteric coated formulations. Aspirin first comes into contact with platelets in the portal circulation, and as a consequence, platelets are exposed to substantially higher drug level than are present in the systemic circulation. Aspirin has a half life of 15-20 minutes in the plasma. Despite rapid clearance of aspirin from the circulation, its antiplatelet effect lasts for the life of platelet owing to the permanent inactivation of a key platelet enzyme, an effect that can only be reversed through the generation of new platelets. Thus there is a complete dissociation between pharmacokinetics and pharmacodynamics of aspirin, allowing the use of a once-a-day regimen for antiplatelet therapy despite the very short half-life of the drug.

By diffusing through the cell membranes, aspirin enters the COX channel, a narrow hydrophobic channel connecting the cell membrane to the catalytic pocket of the enzyme. Aspirin first binds to an arginine-120 residue, a common docking site for all non-steroidal anti-inflammatory drugs. It then acetylates a serine residue (serine 529 in human COX-1 and serine 516 in human COX-2) located in the narrowest section of the channel, thereby preventing arachidonic acid from gaining access to the COX catalytic site of the enzyme [4]. This is an esterification reaction, so the linkage that is formed is covalent. It means that the inhibition is irreversible.

Higher levels of aspirin are needed to inhibit COX-2 than to inhibit COX-1 [5] These differences may account, at least in part, for the need to use considerably higher dose of aspirin to achieve analgesic and anti-inflammatory effects, whereas antiplatelet effects can be obtained with daily doses as low as 30 mg [6].

$$\text{Protein-Serine-}CH_2\text{-OH} + \text{Aspirin} \rightarrow \text{Protein-Serine-}CH_2\text{-O-CO-}CH_3$$

Antiplatelet agents are principally aspirin and clopidogrel, used alone or in combination - have been shown to reduce the formation of fibrin clots by irreversibly inhibiting platelet. Patients who have cardiovascular events like myocardial infarction (MI), ischaemic heart disease, stroke, and unstable angina, non-ST-elevation (NSTE)-acute coronary symdromes (ACS) and ST-elevation MI (STEMI), take aspirin for secondary prevention - that is, to prevent a recurrence. Aspirin also often prescribed for primary prevention, that is, to prevent cardiovascular events in patients with risk factors and is recommended as life-long therapy. Clopidogrel is recommended for periods ranging from 1 to 12 months or as life-long substitute for aspirin in patients in whom aspirin is contraindicated. We shall discuss clopidogrel later in the article. As a result, antiplatelet agents have become essential components of the treatment of these conditions.

The exact time to stop or discontinue antiplatetet therapy prior to surgery or invasive procedure is still controversial. Discontinuation of antiplatelet agents results in recovery of platelet function which contributes to the occurrence of ischaemic events. Unfortunately, neither good evidence from clinical trials nor authoritative guidelines are available to guide physicians faced with this dilemma.

A meta-analysis determined that patients taking aspirin had twice the risk of moderate to severe post-operative complications, although this increase translated only to an increased absolute risk of 2% (1). Most of the centres in the UK recommend discontinuation of aspirin for 7 days prior to the scheduled prostate biopsy. Zhu et al [7] from Denmark also recommended stopping aspirin 1 week prior to all invasive urological procedures. However, there are some published data suggest that aspirin in standard doses do not increase the risk of significant bleeding after prostate biopsy (Table 1 and 2).

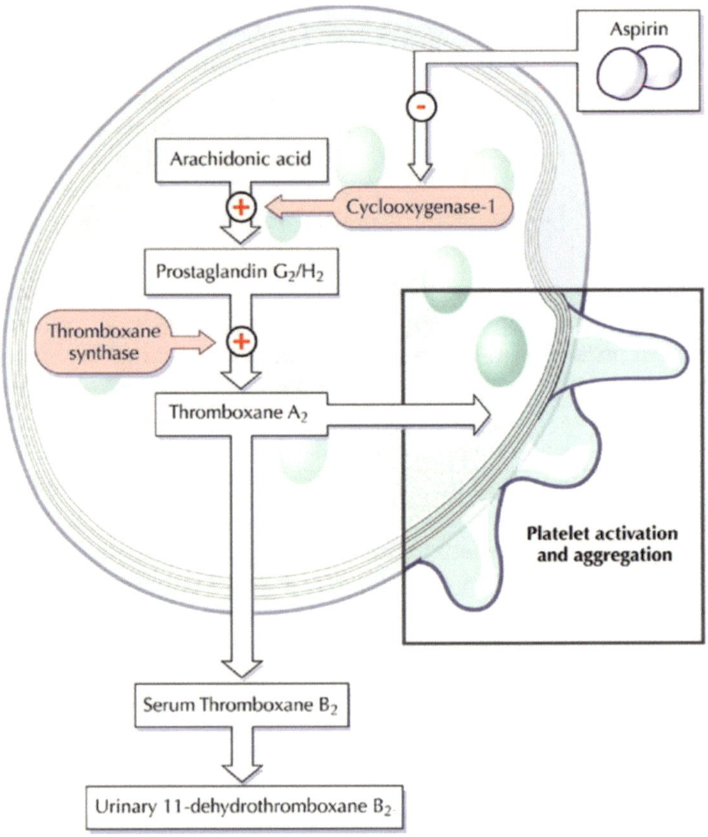

Source: Gasparyan, A. Y. et al. J Am Coll Cardiol 2008;51:1829-1843

Fig. 2. Aspirin inhibition of COX-1 decreases TXA2 production.

In all of the above studies, regarding haemorrhagic complication rates, there were no statistically significant differences between the two groups. Haematuria, rectal bleeding and haemospermia rates between the groups were also comparable. No severe bleeding complications occurred. Some studies showed that an increasing number of cores might increase haemorrhagic events, but it does not affect the duration of bleeding [2,3]. Interestingly, one study showed [9] that aspirin users were significantly older than non-users and haematuria became less likely with increasing age.

There is no guideline on the management of aspirin before taking prostate biopsy. A National Survey performed by Masood et al [12] showed, that only 44% of urology departments have protocols in place relating to aspirin use before prostate biopsy. Of those who replied 65% do not routinely stop aspirin before biopsy. 35% stop aspirin and of these, 52% 1 week before, 41% 2 weeks and 6% >2 weeks before the biopsy. A third of the urologists felt that aspirin increases bleeding complications and 59% stated that the cerebrovascular risks of stopping aspirin outweigh the benefit of stopping aspirin for bleeding.

	Kariotis I et al 2010 [8]	Halliwell OT et al 2008 [9]	Giannarini G et al 2007 [10]	Maan Z 2003 [11]
Study Design	Prospective Questionnaire	Prospective Questionnaire	Prospective Randomized Questionnaire	Prospective cohort Questionnaires
Study Period	Feb 2007 to Sept 2008	2 year	Jan 2005 to Aug 2006	NA
Number of patients/ accessible	530/434	1520/1512	200/196	200/177
aspirin group / non-aspirin /heparin group	152/282/NA	387/1125/NA	67/66/67	36/141/
Number of Biopsy taken	12 cores	NA	10 cores	6 cores
Biopsy needle	18G	NA	18 G	18G
Evaluation time (Questionnaire)	30 day from the date of biopsy	10-14 day from the date of biopsy	14 day post-biopsy	7 day post-biopsy

ASA – acetylsalicylic acid, NA – Not Available

Table 1.

Haemorrhagic Events	Kariotis I et al 2010		Halliwell OT et al 2008		Giannarini G et al 2007			Maan Z 2003	
	ASA	NASA	ASA	NASA	ASA	Hep	NASA	ASA	NASA
Haematuria	64.5%	60.65	72%	61%	78.5%	69.7%	81.5%	56%	59%
Duration of haematuria	4.45 ±2.7	2.4 ± 2.6	4.05	2.85	6	4	2	NA	NA
Rectal Bleeding	33.5%	25.9%	21%	13%	31.3%	29.9%	NA	0%	22%
Duration of rectal bleeding	3.3 ± 1.3	1.9 ± 0.7	2.41	2.03	3	2	1	NA	NA
Haemospermia	90.1%	86.9%	17%	21%	21.4%	18.5%	9.3%	11%	28%
Duration of Haemospermia	21.2 ± 11.9	22.4 ± 10.4	6.8	4.0	NA	NA	NA	NA	NA

Table 2.

A meta-analysis incorporating almost 50,000 patients (14,981 of these on aspirin) found that although aspirin increased the rate of bleeding complications by 1.5 times, it did not lead to greater severity of bleeding complications except for intracranial surgery and possibly TURP [13]

2.1.2 Risk of antiplatelet withdrawal and bridging therapy

There is no doubt that cessation of antiplatelet therapy in patients with a recent coronary stent carries a significant risk [14]. In addition, one French study suggests that recent withdrawal of this therapy may be harmful in patients with coronary artery disease. Half of the withdrawers underwent substitution therapy in the form of non-selective NSAIDS or low molecular weight heparin, which did not protect the patients [15].

2.1.3 Evidences from other specialties

Multiple studies from other specialties have shown the safety of aspirin during a wide array of interventions. Peritoneal dialysis catheter insertion and removal [16], 9-14 gauge core needle breast biopsy [17] and dental extraction [18] all have been shown to be safe with aspirin. Aspirin does not increase the risk for haematoma with spinal or epidural anaesthesia [19], or bleeding with spinal surgery [20].

There are certain clinical instances in which continued aspirin coverage is critical: Aspirin should never be stopped in patients with coronary stents because they face a 45% complication rate and a 20% mortality rate with the highest risk for those with a stent placed in the previous 35 days [21].

2.1.4 Restarting aspirin

A UK National survey [12] reported that the urologists who routinely stop aspirin, the medium (range) time for restarting aspirin after biopsy was 2 (0-10) days.

2.2 Antiplatelet medication – Clopidogrel bisulphate (Plavix, Bristol-Myers Squibb)

Clopidogrel is a thienopyridine that inhibits platelet aggregation by selectively blocking the binding of adenosine diphosphate (ADP) to its platelet receptor, and subsequently ADP-mediated activation of the GP IIb/IIIa complex. ADP stimulates expression of the GP IIb/IIIa receptor and may mediate release of other aggregation agonists and enhance platelet binding of von Willebrand factor. Hence, the end result of ADP inhibition is impairment of platelet aggregation and fibrinogen-mediated platelet crosslinking. Because it irreversibly modifies the platelet ADP receptor, platelets exposed to clopidogrel are affected for the remainder of their life span (7-10 days). After stopping clopidogrel, platelet aggregation and the bleeding times gradually return to baseline value, usually within 5 days.

Clopidogrel has a mixed safety record depending on which intervention is studied. It does not increase the risk of haematoma with spinal anaesthesia [22]. The maintenance of clopidogrel during surgery or invasive procedures has not been extensively studied. Patients taking clopidogrel after coronary artery intervention have a high risk of late stent thrombosis if they interrupt their medications (usually clopidogrel & aspirin). Of patients who stopped medications prematurely, 29% suffered stent thrombosis and 45% of those patients died [23]. There have been several non-urological studies assessing the risk of bleeding in patients on clopidogrel undergoing cardiothoracic surgery [24], plastic surgery [25], ophthalmology [26] and vascular surgery [27]. However, conclusions regarding the risk of bleeding are contradictory. To date, there have been very few reports

in the urological literature regarding the risks associated with clopidogrel continuation and urological surgery.
A UK survey [28] on the peri-operative management of Urological patients with clopidogrel showed that majority of the urologists stop clopidogrel prior to TUR surgery (96.6%), major urological surgery (91.7%), TRUS Biopsy (90.6%), ESWL (81.8%), and Cystoscopy & Biopsy (70.1%). Almost half of the respondents (total 570 respondents) would stop aspirin irrespective of its indication and 40.7% never consulted a cardiologist/haematologist before stopping clopidogrel. Over half (55%) reported bleeding complications in patients who continued clopidogrel during interventions and 7.4% responders reported an adverse thrombotic event after discontinuing the drug.

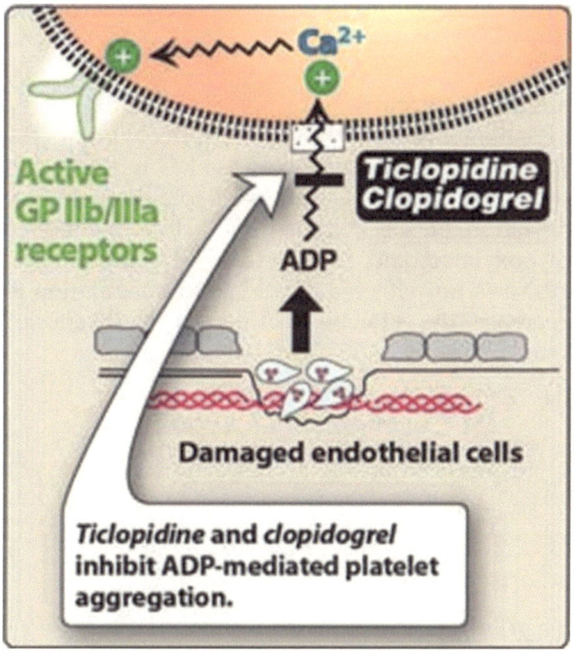

Fig. 3. Pathway of blockage of ADP receptors by clopidogrel. Source: Harvey, R; Champe, P "Lippincott illustrated reviews: Pharmacology", 4th edition. LWW: 2009.

2.2.1 Bridging therapy

If patients take aspirin in addition to clopidogrel because of a coronary artery stent, the aspirin should be continued to mitigate the risk of late stent thrombosis [29] and clopidogrel should be restarted following TRUS biopsy as soon as possible using a loading dose. Bridging anticoagulation for patients who must interrupt clopidogrel is controvertial. Anticoagulation with warfarin or heparin has not proven useful [30] and is questionable [31]. In general, antiplatelet therapy should not be interrupted until patients are beyond the safety window. If an intervention cannot be delayed, the risks of drug interruption should be weighed carefully against the risk of bleeding. As a practical matter, the surgeon, cardiologist, haematologist and anaesthesiologist should consult on each case regarding the risk of peri-operative bleeding if antiplatelet therapy is continued and the risk of ischaemic events if therapy is discontinued. If the course is not acceptable, postponement of the surgery should be considered if possible.

2.2.2 Re-starting clopidogrel

The decision of each patient should be individualised based on the clinical situation. An attempt should be made to restart the clopidogrel as soon as possible after the procedure, when the risk of bleeding is minimal, to minimise the risk of thrombo-embolic phenomena. It should be restarted using a loading dose.

2.3 Warfarin (4-hydroxycoumarins)

Warfarin inhibits the formation of vitamin K-dependent coagulation proteins, i.e., factor II, VII, IX, X and protein C and S. These are proteins of the extrinsic pathway and thus would be monitored by INR. These diminished factors lead to decreased fibrin clot formation and, to a lesser extent, primary haemostasis by platelets (because thrombin is an important activator of platelets).

2.3.1 Mechanism of action of warfarin

Warfarin is a vitamin K antagonist. It produces its anticoagulant effect by interfering with the vitamin K cycle. Specifically, it interacts with the KO reductase enzyme so that vitamin KO cannot be recycled back to vitamin K. This leads to a depletion of vitamin KH_2, thereby limiting the γ- carboxylation of the coagulation factors mentioned above. Factors like prothrombin are not carboxylated, and cannot effectively bind to phospholipid membranes. Its activation by Factor Xa is not affected. Thus blood coagulation is limited. Therapeutic doses of warfarin decrease the effects of Vitamin K-dependant clotting factors by approximately 30 to 40%.

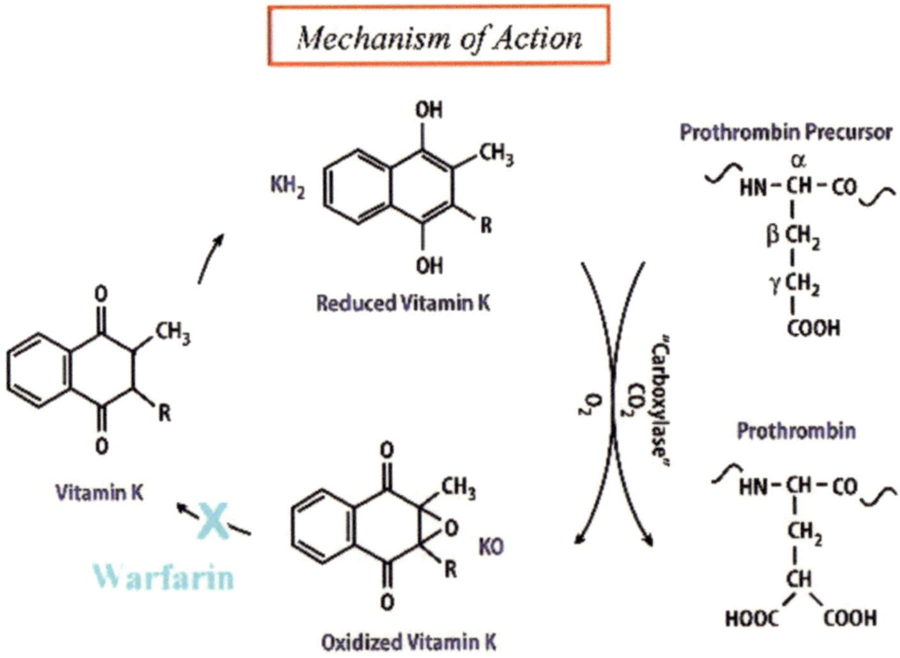

Fig. 4. The carboxylation process is associated with the vitamin K cycle. In this cycle, vitamin K is reduced by enzyme Vitamin K reductase to its hydroquinone form, vitamin KH_2, which then catalyses the carboxylation process and is converted to its epoxide (vitamin KO). This is then converted back to vitamin K by the enzyme Vitamin KO reductase.

2.3.2 Bleeding risks during invasive procedures

Bleeding is the obvious risk when continuing warfarin during surgical interventions. One study found a seven fold increase in moderate to severe post-operative complications in patients taking the medication [32].

The relation between warfarin use and the frequency of bleeding complications after TRUS biopsy was reported in a prospective study of 1000 patients. Forty nine patients continuously used warfarin before and after the biopsy. The prevalence and severity of bleeding complications were assessed by a questionnaire 10 days after the biopsy. There were no significant difference in the severity of bleeding between patients taking warfarin and controls [28]. However, limitations of this study include non-randomized design, patients had either 4 or 6 core biopsies and complications were entered retrospectively 10 days after biopsy.

Some studies showed that maintaining a therapeutic level of warfarin anticoagulation is safe for many interventions. Ihezu et al [33] showed less bleeding in patient taking warfarin with an average INR of 2.2, than in control subject. Similar evidences are found in some non-urological invasive interventions - trans-femoral coronary angiography using 5 or 6 French sheaths [INR 2.0-3.0] [34], cataract surgery [35], dental surgery [INR upto 4.2] [36], and dermatologic surgery [INR upto 4.5] [37].

A survey among urologists and radiologists found that 84% of urologists stopped it 4 days before TRUS biopsy and 95% of radiologists stopped it 5 days before TRUS biopsy. An international normalized ratio below 1.5 is accepted for most elective procedures [38].

2.3.3 Bridging therapy and risk of warfarin withdrawal

The decision whether to stop anticoagulants depends on the indications for anticoagulation and the risk of thrombosis in a particular patient. The decision should be discussed with the patient and the primary physician managing the anticoagulant. Several regimens have been developed to increase the safety of warfarin interruption. The simplest involves stopping the medication 3-5 days before the intervention and restarting it immediately afterwards [38]. An anticoagulation effect generally occurs within 24 hours after the drug administration, though peak anticoagulant effect may be delayed 72 to 96 hours. The action of a single dose of warfarin lasts 2 to 5 days, & the effects of warfarin may become more pronounced as effects of daily doses overlap.

An alternative regimen is to reduce the warfarin dose to achieve an INR of 1.5-2.0 for surgery or interventions [38]. Bridging anticoagulation with unfractionated heparin or low-molecular weight heparin (LMWH) should be considered for patients at the highest risk of thromboembolism, such as those with prosthetic metallic heart valves. This involves stopping warfarin 3-5 days before the surgery and administering unfractionated heparin or LMWH until 6-24 hours before the procedure [38].

Heparin, containing the unique five-residue sequence, forms a high-affinity complex with antithrombin. The formation of antithrombin - heparin complex greatly increases the rate of inhibition of two principle procoagulant proteases, factor Xa and thrombin. The normally slow rate of inhibition of both these enzymes (~ 10^3 - 10^4 $M^{-1}s^{-1}$) by antithrombin alone (see graph below) is increased about a 1,000-fold by heparin. Accelerated inactivation of both the active forms of proteases prevents the subsequent conversion of fibrinogen to fibrin that is crucial for clot formation.

On the other hand, compared with the unfractionated heparin, low-molecular weight heparin has a greater ratio of anti-factor Xa / anti-factor IIa activity, greater bioavailabity, and longer duration of action. It is also suitable as outpatient treatment and requires less monitoring [39]. It does not cross placenta, therefore it can be used during pregnancy.

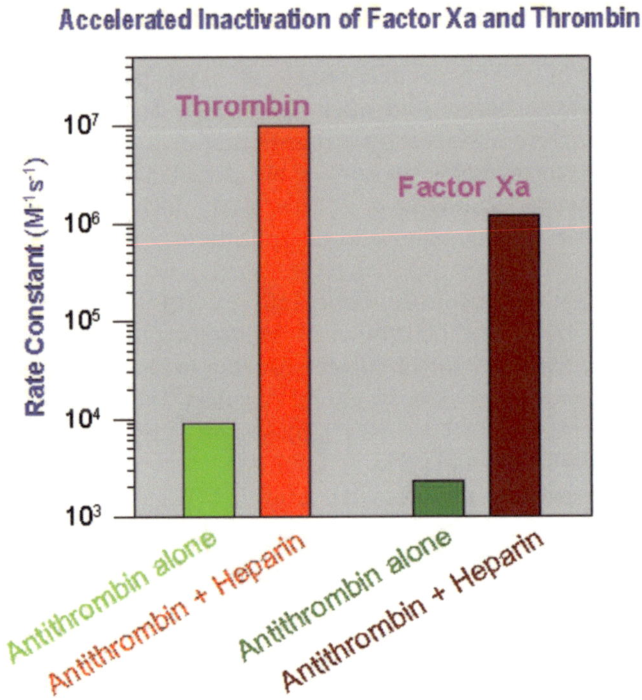

Graph: Effect of action of heparin

Patients with an acute venous thromboembolism in the previous 3 months or an arterial embolism in the previous month should receive unfractionated heparin or LMWH. The risk for recurrent venous thromboembolism is high [40] if anticoagulation is stopped in the first month after an acute event (40%), and decreases if the anticoagulants are not stopped until the second or third month (10%). The bridging anticoagulant is usually restarted as soon after the procedure as is considered safe to do so and continued until a therapeutic INR has been established with warfarin.

3. Other inherent bleeding risks

Identification of patients at high risk for bleeding is the first step in managing those on antiplatelet agents or warfarin who require invasive procedures. Demographic factors that increase the likelihood of bleeding are advanced age, previous history of bleeding events, haemorrhagic peptic ulcer or haemorrhagic stroke [31]. Medical conditions that increase the risks of bleeding include obesity, diabetes, hypertension, renal impairment, heart failure, other major organ dysfunction and haemostatic disorders [31, 41]. Patients with these conditions present a particularly difficult dilemma for clinicians. Data on patients with these conditions are not found in the medical literature. A unified validated method of sorting patients in terms of their bleeding risk and weighing it against their risk of ischaemic events is sorely needed but is yet unavailable.

4. Comment

There is insufficient clinical evidence to establish comprehensive guidelines regarding continuation of aspirin during TRUS biopsy. However, data are emerging and from some level 2 evidence it appears that patients on ASA should have this maintained during TRUS biopsy. In clearly identified cases, where bleeding might threaten the patient's life e.g. after acute cardiac events, the discontinuation protocol must be established in conjunction with cardiologist and the ASA therapy resumed as soon as possible. Bridging with LMWH is not recommended in the aspirin or clopidogrel group. Consideration should be given to postponing TRUS biopsy in high risk individuals. Patients with combination of aspirin and clopidogrel should at least continue aspirin during the procedure. Evidence on discontinuation of warfarin is sparse but emerging. However, bridging therapy with heparin in this situation could be an effective replacement of warfarin. There is an urgent need for research in order to change the practice of stopping anticoagulants and to establish a comprehensive set of recommendation before the TRUS biopsy.

5. References

[1] Rodriguez LV, Terris MK. Risks and complications of transrectal ultrasound guided prostate biopsy: A prospective study and review of literature. J Urol 1998; 160:2115-20.
[2] Ghani KR, Dundas D, Patel U. Bleeding after transrectal ultrasonography-guided prostate biopsy: a study of 7-day morbidity after a six, eight, and 12 core biopsy protocol. BJU Intl 2004; 94:1014-20
[3] Naughton CK, Ornstein DK, Smith DS, Catalona WJ. Pain and morbidity of transrectal ultrasound guided prostate biopsy: A prospective randomized trial of 6 versus 12 cores. J Urol 2000; 163: 168-71.
[4] Loll PJ, Picot D, Garavito RM. "The structural basis of aspirin activity inferred from the crystal structure of inactivated prostaglandin H2 synthase. Nat Struct Biol 1995; 2: 637-43.
[5] Cipollone F, Patrignani P, Greco A, et al. "Differential suppression of thromboxane biosynthesis by indobufen and aspirin in patients with unstable angina". Circulation 1997;96:1109-16.
[6] Patrono C, Coller B, FitzGerald GA, Hirsh J, Roth G. "Platelet-active drugs: the relationship among dose, effectiveness, and side effects: the Seventh ACCP Conference on Antithrombotic and Thrombolytic Therapy". Chest 2004; 126: Suppl: 234S-264S.
[7] Zhu JP, Davidsen MB, Meyhoff HH. Aspirin, a silent, risk factor in urology. Scand J Urol Nephrol 1995; 29: 369-374.
[8] Kariotis I, Philippou P, Volanis D, Serafetinides E, Delakas D. Safety of ultrasound-guided transrectal extended prostate biopsy in patients receiving low-dose aspirin. Int Braz J Urol 2010 May-June; 36(3): 308-16.
[9] Halliwell OT, Yadegafar G, Lane C, Dewbury KC. Transrectal ultrasound guided biopsy of the prostate: aspirin increases the incidence of minor bleeding complications. Clin Radiol. 2008 May ; 63(5): 557-61

[10] Giannarini G, Mogorovich A, Valent F, Morelli G, De Maria M, Manassero F, Barbone F, Selli C. Continuing or discontinuing low-dose aspirin before transrectal prostate biopsy: results of prospective randomized trial. Urology. 2007 Sept; 70(3): 501-5.

[11] Maan Z, Cutting CW, Patel U, Kerry S, Pietrzak P, Perry MJ, Kirby RS. Morbidity of transrectal ultrasonography-guided prostate biopsies in patients after the continued use of low-dose aspirin. BJU Int. 2003 Jun; 91(9): 798-800.

[12] Junaid Masood, Azhar Hafeez, John Calleary and Jayanta M. Barua. Aspirin use and transrectal ultrasounography-guided prostate biopsy: A National Survey. BJU Int. 2007. 99, 965-971.

[13] Burger W, Chemnitius JM, Kneissl GD, Rucker G. *Low dose aspirin for secondary cardiovascular prevention – cardiovascular risks after its perioperative withdrawal versus bleeding risks with its continuation – review and meta-analysis.* J Intern Med 2005; 399-414.

[14] Pompa JJ, Berger P, Ohman EM, Harrington RA, Grines C, Weitz JI: Antithrombotic therapy during percutaneous coronary intervention; the seventh ACCP Conference on Antithrombotic and thrombolytic therapy. Chest 2004; 126: 576S-599S.

[15] Collet JP, Montalescot G, Blanchet B, et al. Impact of prior use of recent withdrawal of oral antiplatelet agents on acute coronary syndromes. Circulation 2004; 110: 2361-2367.

[16] Shpitz B, Plotkin E, Spindel Z, et al. Should aspirin therapy be withheld before insertion and/or removal of a permanent peritoneal dialysis catheter? *Am Surg* 2002;68 : 762–764

[17] Somerville P, Seifert PJ, Destounis SV, Murphy PF, Young W. Anticoagulation and bleeding risk after core needle biopsy. *AJR* 2008; 191:1194 –1197.

[18] Aframian DJ, Lalla RV, Peterson DE. Management of dental patients taking common hemostasis-altering medications. *Oral Surg Oral Med Oral Pathol Oral Radiol Endod* 2007;103 [suppl]: S45 e1–S45 e11.

[19] Horlocker TT, Wedel DJ, Schroeder DR, et al. Preoperative antiplatelet therapy does not increase the risk of spinal hematoma associated with regional anesthesia. *Anesth Analg*1995; 80:303 –309.

[20] West SW, Otley CC, Nguyen TH, et al. Cutaneous surgeons cannot predict blood-thinner status by intraoperative visual inspection. *Plast Reconstr Surg* 2002;110 : 98–103.

[21] Vicenzi MN, Meislitzer T, Heitzinger B, Halaj M, Fleisher LA, Metzler H. Coronary artery stenting and non-cardiac surgery: a prospective outcome study. *Br J Anaesth* 2006;96 : 686–693.

[22] Harder S, Klinkhardt U, Alvarez JM. Avoidance of bleeding during surgery in patients receiving anticoagulant and/or antiplatelet therapy: pharmacokinetic and pharmacodynamic considerations. *Clin Pharmacokinet* 2004; 43:963 –981.

[23] Iakovou I, Schmidt T, Bonizzoni E, et al. Incidence, predictors, and outcome of thrombosis after successful implantation of drug-eluting stents. *JAMA* 2005;293 :2126 –2130.

[24] Yende S, Wunderink RG. Effect of clopidogrel on bleeding after coronary artery bypass surgery. *Crit Care Med.* 2001;29:2271–5.

[25] Kovich O, Otley CC. Perioperative management of anticoagulants and platelet inhibitors for cutaneous surgery: a survey of current practice. *Dermatol Surg.* 2002;28:513–7.

[26] Davies BR. Combined aspirin and clopidogrel in cataract surgical patients: a new risk factor for ocular haemorrhage? *Br J Ophthalmol.* 2004;88:1226–7.

[27] Smout J, Stansby G. Current practice in the use of antiplatelet agents in the peri-operative period by UK vascular surgeons. *Ann R Coll Surg Engl.* 2003;85:97–101.

[28] Gaurav Mukerji, Indumina Munasinghe, and Asif Raza. A Survey of the Peri-operative Management of Urological Patients on Clopidogrel. Ann R Coll Surg Engl. 2009 May; 91(4): 313-320.

[29] Chassot PG, Delabays A, Spahn DR. Perioperative antiplatelet therapy: the case for continuing therapy in patients at risk of myocardial infarction. *Br J Anaesth* 2007;99 : 316–328.

[30] Grines CL, Bonow RO, Casey DE, et al. Prevention of premature discontinuation of dual antiplatelet therapy in patients with coronary artery stents: a science advisory from the American Heart Association, American College of Cardiology, Society for Cardiovascular Angiography and Interventions, American College of Surgeons, and American Dental Association, with representation from the American College of Physicians. *Circulation* 2007;115 : 813–818.

[31] ColletJP, Montalescot G. *Premature withdrawal and alternative therapies to dual oral antiplatelet therapy. Eur Heart J (2006) 8(Suppl. G):*G46–G52.

[32] Chassot PG, Delabays A, Spahn DR. Perioperative use of anti-platelet drugs. *Best Pract Res Clin Anaesthesiol*2007; 21:241 –256.

[33] Ihezue CU, Smart J, Dewbury KC, et al. Biopsy of the prostate guided by transrectal ultrasound: relation between warfarin use and incidence of bleeding complications. Clin Radiol 2005; 60: 459-63.

[34] El-Jack SS, Ruygrok PN, Webster MW, et al. Effectiveness of manual pressure hemostasis following transfemoral coronary angiography in patients on therapeutic warfarin anticoagulation. *Am J Cardiol*2006; 97:485 –488.

[35] Dunn AS, Turpie AG. Perioperative management of patients receiving oral anticoagulants: a systematic review. *Arch Intern Med* 2003; 163:901 –908.

[36] Jeske AH, Suchko GD. Lack of a scientific basis for routine discontinuation of oral anticoagulation therapy before dental treatment. *J Am Dent Assoc* 2003;134 :1492 –1497.

[37] Blasdale C, Lawrence CM. Perioperative international normalized ratio level is a poor predictor of postoperative bleeding complications in dermatological surgery patients taking warfarin. *Br J Dermatol* 2008; 158:522 –526.

[38] Kearon C, Hirsh J. Management of anticoagulation before and after elective surgery. N Engl J Med 1997; 336: 1506-11.

[39] Larson BJ, Zumberg MS, Kitchens CS. A feasibility study of continuing dose-reduced warfarin for invasive procedures in patients with high thromboembolic risk. *Chest* 2005;127 : 922–927.

[40] Douketis JD, Johnson JA, Turpie AG. Low-molecular-weight heparin as bridging anticoagulation during interruption of warfarin: assessment of a standardized periprocedural anticoagulation regimen. *Arch Intern Med* 2004; 164:1319 -1326.
[41] EikelboomJW, Hirsh J. *Bleeding and management of bleeding. Eur Heart J (2006) 8(Suppl. G):G38–G45.*

7

Malignant Transformation and Stromal Invasion from Normal Appearing Prostate Tissues: True or False?

Yan-gao Man
The Diagnostic and Translational Research Center
Henry Jackson Foundation, Gaithersburg
USA

1. Introduction

The human prostate epithelium, which is the histological origin of most prostate malignancies, is physically separated from the stroma by a layer of basal cells and the basement membrane. Basal cells are inter-connected by intercellular junctions and adhesion molecules, constituting a continuous sheet encircling luminal cells [1-2]. The basement membrane is composed of type IV collagen, laminins, and other molecules, forming a continuous lining surrounding and attaching to the basal cell layer [3-4] (Fig 1). The basement membrane and the basal cell layer are intermixed to form a dense fibrous capsule surrounding all epithelial cells. Due to these relationships, disruption of the basal cell layer and the basement membrane is a pre-requisite for tumor invasion or metastasis.

It is a commonly held belief that prostate carcinogenesis progresses sequentially from normal to hyperplasia, to prostatic intraepithelial neoplasia (PIN), and to invasive or metastatic lesions [5-8]. Progression from PIN to invasion is believed to be triggered by overproduction of proteolytic enzymes primarily by cancer cells, which cause degradation of the tumor capsule [9-10]. These theories are consistent with laboratory findings from cell cultures and animal models, whereas are hard to reconcile with a number of critical facts. **First,** previous studies revealed that some healthy men between 19 and 29 years old had a spectrum of proliferative lesions, including hyperplasia, PIN, and incipient adenocarcinoma [11-13]. **Second**, recent studies have detected a DNA phenotype identical to that of invasive prostate cancer in some "healthy" men, and also in normal prostate tissues adjacent to prostate cancer [14-17]. **Third**, a majority of PIN express high levels of proteolytic enzymes, but only 10-30% of untreated PIN progress to invasive lesions during patients' lifetime [18-21]. **Fourth**, cancer of unknown primary site is one of the 10 most frequent cancers worldwide and the 4th most common cause of cancer deaths [22-24].

Together, these facts argue that the linear model of carcinogenesis [5-8] and enzyme theory of tumor invasion [9-10] are not universally applicable to all prostate cancer cases. These facts also suggest that the past efforts to classify tumor progression and invasion purely based on the profiles of epithelial cells may have overlooked some essential factors. As over 90% of prostate cancer related mortality result from invasion related diseases, and the incidence of PIN could be up to 16.5%-25% in prostate biopsies [25-27], there is an urgent need to uncover the intrinsic mechanism of tumor invasion and to distinguish aggressive and indolent PIN for optimal or personalized treatment. Unfortunately, none of the current approaches could predict which PIN lesions will progress [28-31]. The only established approach to monitor PIN progression is repeat biopsy [28-31], which is costly and painful.

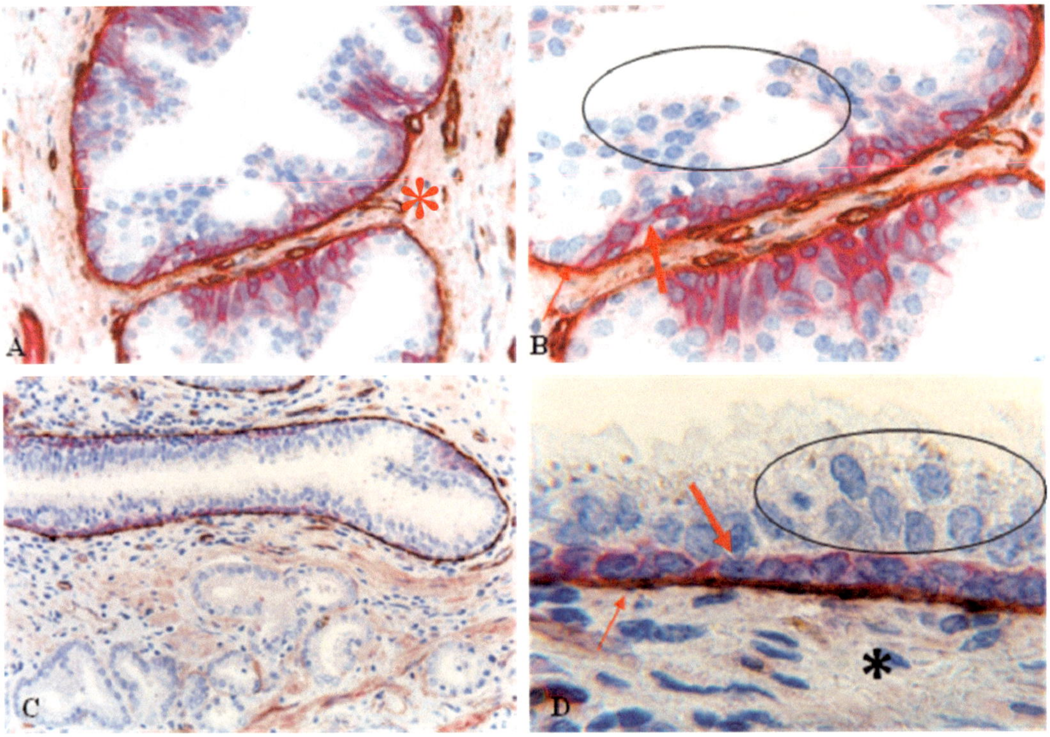

Fig. 1. Structural relationships among the epithelium (circles), basal cell layer (thick arrows), basement membrane (thin arrows), and stroma (asterisks). Human prostate tissue sections were double immunostained for collagen IV (brown) and cytokeratin 34βE12 (red). A and C: 150X. B and D: a higher (500X) magnification of A and C.

Promoted by the fact that the basal cell layer is the sole source of tumor suppressor p63 and maspin [32-35], and that degradation of the basal cell layers is a pre-requisite for tumor invasion, our resent studies have attempted to identify early signs of basal cell degradation. Our initial study examined the physical integrity of the basal cell layers in 50 patients with co-existing pre-invasive and invasive prostate tumors. Of 2,047 ducts and acini examined, 197 were found to harbor focal disruptions (the absence of basal cells resulting in a gap greater than the combined size of at least 3 basal cells) in their basal cell layers. The frequency of focal basal cell layer disruptions (FBCLD) varied from none in 22 (44%) cases to over 1/3 of the ducts or acini with FBCLD in 17 (34%) cases (Table 1) [36]. Of the 17 cases with a high frequency of FBCLD, 5 harbored large acinar or duct clusters that are morphologically normal in H& E stained sections, but all harbored focal disruptions in the surrounding capsule in immunostained sections. As shown in Fig 2a, each of the 12 epithelial structures in one of such cases harbors FBCLD, but none of the 12 morphologically similar epithelial structures in Case B shows FBCLD.

Case number	No disruptions	< 30% disruptions	≥ 30% disruptions	p
50	22 (44%)	11 (22%)	17 (34%)	< 0.01

Table 1. Frequencies of focal basal cell layer disruptions among cases

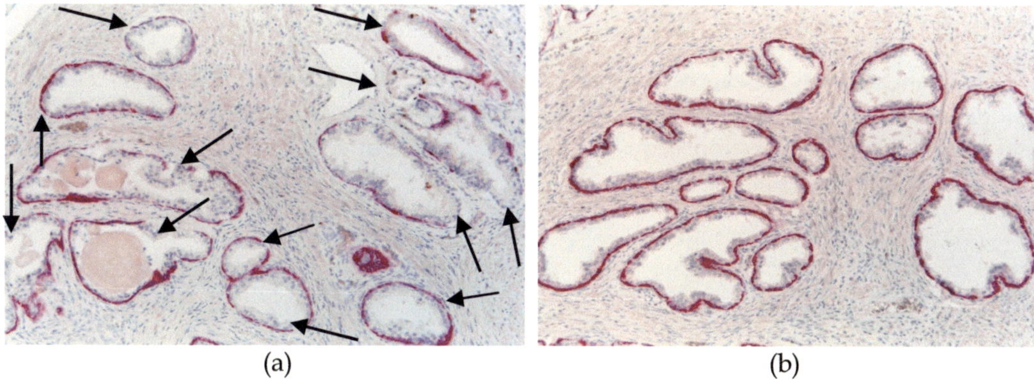

Fig. 2. Different frequencies of FBCLD among cases. Double immunostained for CK 34ßE12 (red) and Ki-67 (brown). In Case A, all 12 epithelial structures show FBCLD (arrows), whereas in Case B, none shows FBCLD. 200X.

Compared to their non-disrupted counterpart, focally disrupted basal cell layers in these 17 cases displayed several unique alterations that were not or rarely seen in morphologically similar structures in other cases [36-44]:

A. significantly reduced expression of tumor suppressor p63: In sections double immunostained for p63 and CK 34βE12, an average of 87% of the basal cells in non-disrupted layers expressed both molecules, while only 59% of the basal cells in focally disrupted layers showed p63 expression (Fig 3; Table 2).

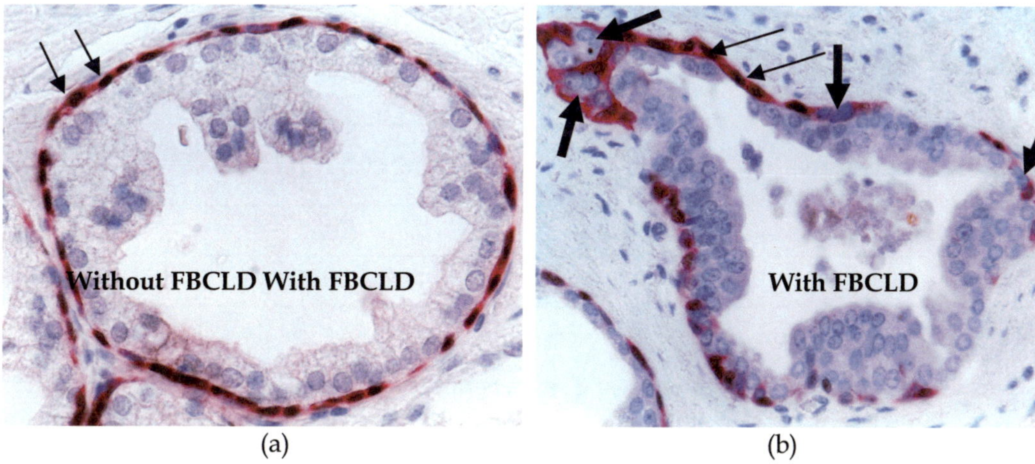

Fig. 3. Reduction of p63 expression in focally disrupted basal cell layers. Sections were double immunostained for CK 34ßE12 (red) and p63 (black). Thin and thick arrows identify cells with and without p63 expression, respectively. 400X.

Basal cell layer status	Number of ducts or acini	Percentage of p63 (+) cells	P
With disruption	197	59%	
W/o disruption	197	87%	< 0.01

Table 2. p63 expression in basal cell layers with and without focal disruption

B. significantly reduced expression of proliferating cell nuclear antigen (PCNA): In sections double immunostained for PCNA and CK34βE12, an average of 74% of the normal basal cells showed PCNA expression, but only 51% of basal cells in disrupted basal layers showed PCNA expression (Fig. 4; Table 3).

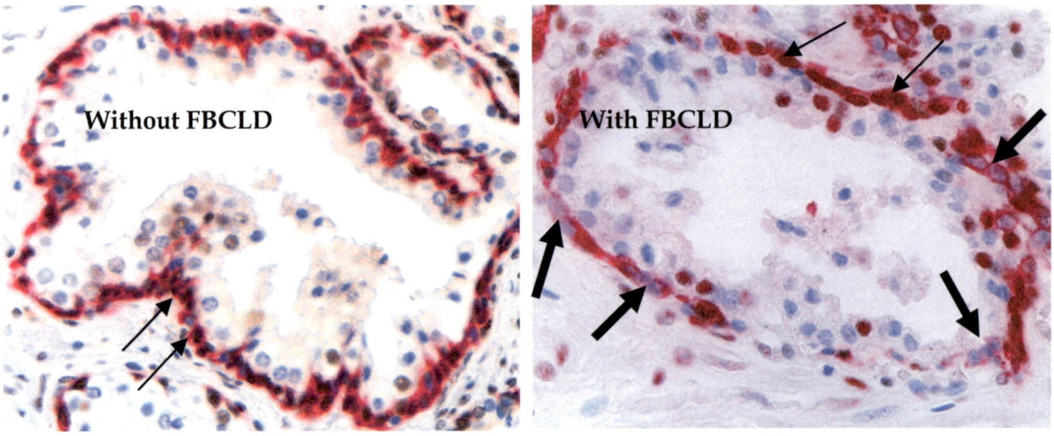

Fig. 4. Significantly reduced PCNA expression in basal cell layers with FBCLD. Double immunostained for CK34 βE12 (red) and PCNA (black). Thin and thick arrows identify basal cells with and without PCNA expression, respectively. 400X

Basal cell layer status	Number of ducts or acini	% of PCNA (+) cells	P
With disruption	50	51%	
W/o disruption	50	74%	< 0.01

Table 3. PCNA expression in basal cell layers with and without focal disruption

C. significantly elevated apoptosis and degeneration: Of 78 epithelial structures with FBCLD examined, 59 (75.6%) harbored apoptotic basal cells, compared to 9% (11.5%) in 78 similar structures with intact basal layers.

Under high magnification, basal cells near FBCLD often had cytological signs of degeneration, including nuclear swelling, shrinkage, fragmentation, or rod-like structures of fused basal cells (Fig. 5).

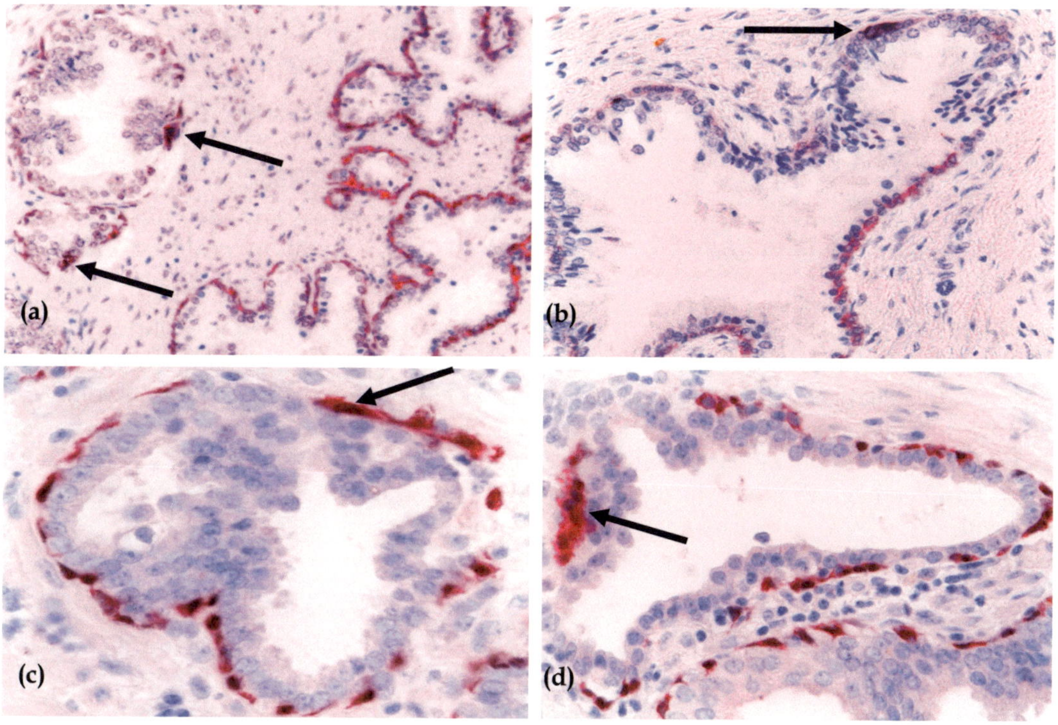

Fig. 5. Elevated apoptosis and degeneration in focally disrupted basal cell layers. Section was assessed for apoptosis (a-b) or CK34βE12 expression (c-d). Arrows identify apoptotic or degenerated basal cells arranged as rod-like structures. 300X.

D. significantly elevated leukocyte infiltration: In sections double immunostained for CK 34βE12 and leukocyte common antigen (LCA), most structures with FBCLD showed leukocyte infiltration, but most structures with non-disrupted layers had no leukocyte infiltration (Table 4). Most leukocytes were located near FBCLD (Fig 6).

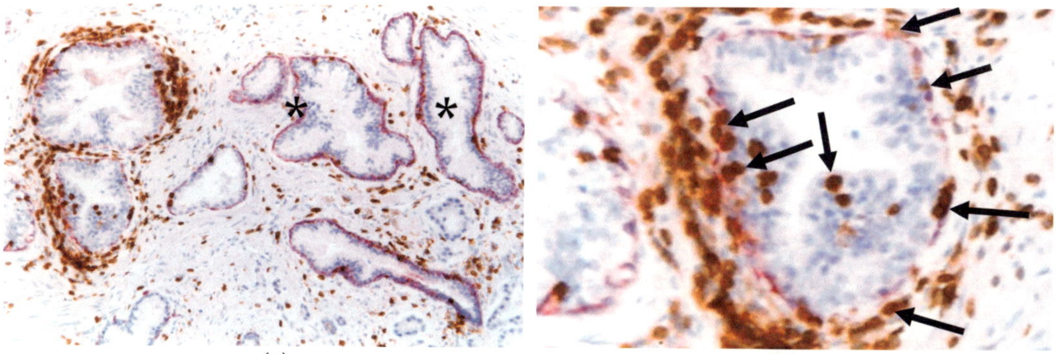

(a) (b)

Fig. 6. FBCLD and infiltration of LCA=positive cells. Double immunostained for CK34βE12 (red) and LCA (brown). Arrows identify infiltrates within the epithelium or near FBCLD. No leukocyte infiltration was seen in ducts with non-disrupted basal cell layers (asterisks). A; 100X. B: a higher (300X) magnification of A.

Basal cell layer status	Number of ducts or acini	Number of leukocyte infiltration	P
With focal disruptions	201	183 (91.0%)	< 0.01
Without focal disruptions	201	67 (33.3%)	

Table 4. Leukocyte infiltration in epithelial structures with and without focal basal cell layer disruption

E. a total loss of the expression of all basal cell phenotypic markers: In addition to focal alterations, the entire basal cell layer in some epithelial structures of some cases showed degenerative changes. These basal cell layers were morphologically distinct, surrounding PIN or normal-appearing duct or acinar clusters (Fig 7). All the basal cells, however, lacked the expression of basal cell specific markers (Fig 7). Epithelial associated with these basal cell layers often showed malignant cytology, including enlarged nuclei and nucleoli.

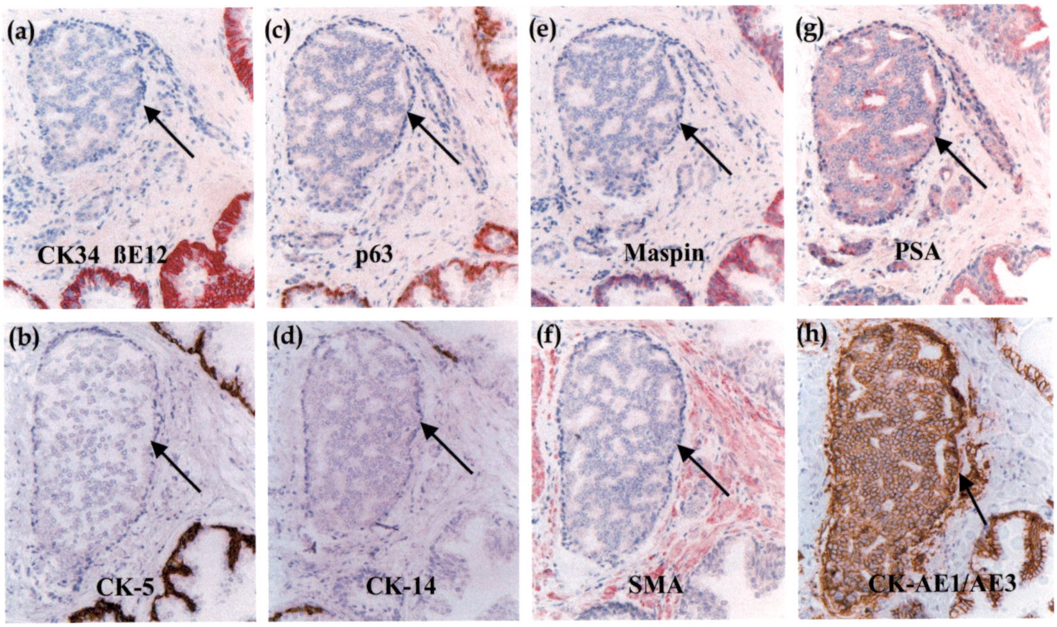

Fig. 7. Morphologically distinct basal cell layers lack expression of all basal cell specific markers. Immunostained for basal (a-e), stromal (f), and epithelial (g-h) cell markers. Arrows identify altered basal cell layers. 200X.

In addition, these basal cell layers were devoid of expression of PCNA, in contrast to normal basal cells and associated tumor cells, which were strongly positive for PCNA (Fig. 8). Epithelial structures with altered basal cell layers often had mast cell infiltration, which was not seen in structures with intact basal cell layers (Fig 8).

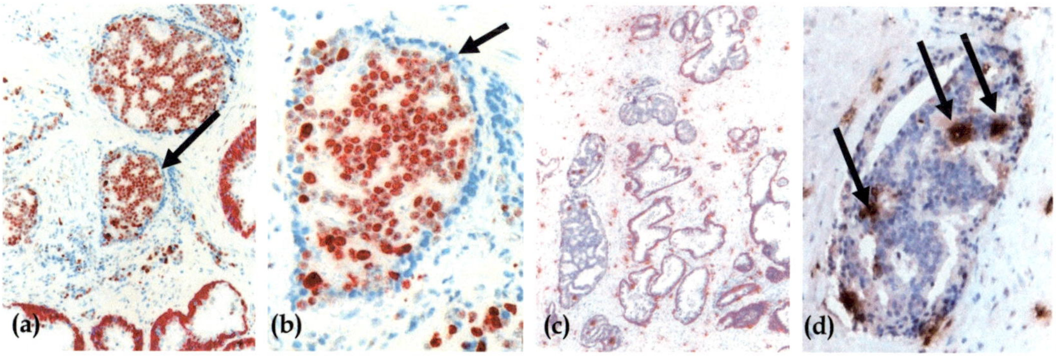

Fig. 8. PNA expression and mast cell infiltration in acini with altered basal cell layers. Double immunostained for CK34 βE12 (red) and PCNA (brown) or mast cells (black). Arrows identify basal cells or mast cells. a & c: 100X. b & d: 400X.

Together, these findings suggest that focally disrupted basal cell layers are likely to be under degeneration. As the basal cell layer is the sole source of several tumor suppressors [29-32], degenerated basal cells are very likely to have impaired or reduced paracrine inhibitory functions on tumor cell growth and invasion. In contrast to degenerative alterations in basal cells, luminal cells overlying FBCLD showed several signs of proliferative alterations that were not seen in their adjacent counterparts distant from the disruptions:

A. significantly elevated proliferation: In section double immunostained for basal cell and proliferation markers, epithelial structures with FBCLD had a significantly higher proliferation index than their morphologically similar counterparts without FBCLD, and most proliferating cells were located at or near FBCLD (Fig.9; Table 5).

Duct or acinar type	Total number	With proliferating cells	P
With disruption	78	47 (62.5%)	< 0.01
W/o disruption	78	8 (10.2%)	

Table 5. Cell proliferation in epithelial structures with and without focal basal cell layer disruption

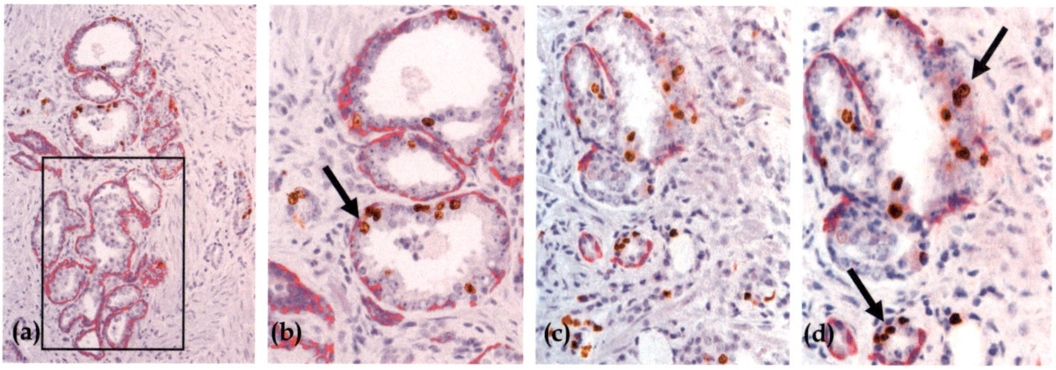

Fig. 9. Increased proliferation in ducts with FBCLD. Sections were double immunostained for CK 34βE12 (red) and Ki-67 (brown). Arrows identify proliferating cell clusters. Note that in a-b, KI-67 positive cells are seen in ducts with FBCLD, but not in adjacent ducts without FBCLD (square). a & c: 100X. b & d: a higher (400X) magnification of a and c, respectively.

B. significantly higher expression of malignancy- and tumor invasion-related molecules: Elevated expression of prostate specific antigen (PSA) and alpha-methylacyl-CoA racemase (AMACR), are seen in cells overlying FBCLD (Fig.10a & b), and also in normal ducts lacked the expression of basal cell markers (Fig. 10c & d). In contrast, cells within the same duct, and adjacent ducts with intact basal cell layers were negative (Fig 10).

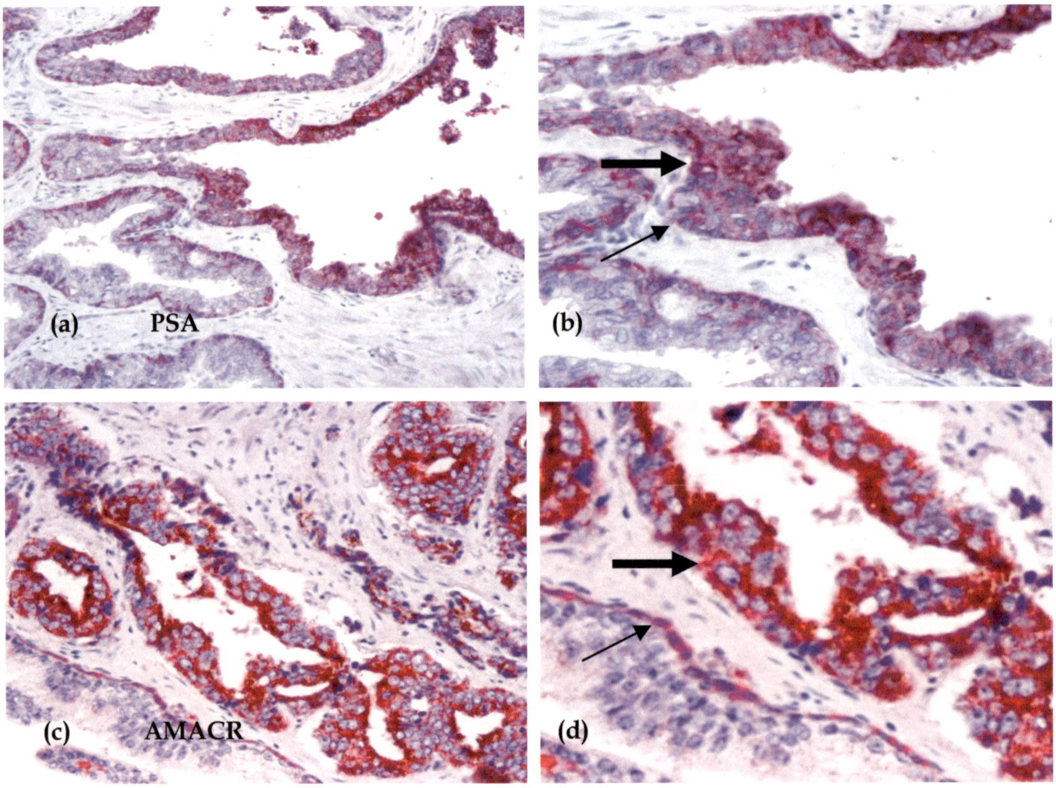

Fig. 10. PSA and AMACR expression in cells overlying FBCLD and ducts with altered basal cells. Double immunostained for CK34 βE12 (red) and PSA or AMACR (brown). Thick arrows identify cells with AMACR or PSA expression. Thin arrows identify residual basal cells. a & c: 100X. b & d: a higher magnification (400X) of a & c, respectively.

C. physical continuity with, and morphological resemblance to, invasive prostate cancer: A vast majority of these normal appearing acinar or duct clusters were immediately adjacent to, or blended with, invasive cancers. In some cases, cells overlying FBCLD had significantly enlarged nuclei and nucleoli, and were often in physical continuity with, or morphologically similar to, their adjacent invasive counterparts (Fig 11).

In some cases, multiple epithelial cell nests appeared to be "budding" from the same acinus or duct (Fig.12). These "budding" cells had a higher proliferation and were similar to adjacent invasive cancer cells. The only difference was that "budding" cells are often associated with residual basal cells (Fig 12, thin arrows).

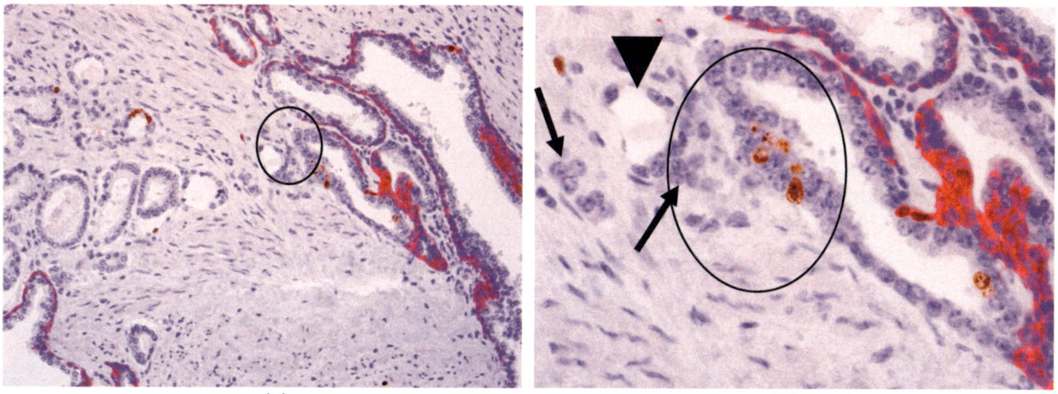

(a) (b)

Fig. 11. Physical continuity with, and morphological resemblance to, invasive cancer. Double immunostained for CK 34ßE12 (red) and Ki-67 (brown). Circles identify proliferating cells overlying FBCLD. Note that cells overlying FBCLD are in direct continuity and similar to invasive cancer cells (arrows). Cells near FBCLD appear to invade a small and dilated vein (arrowhead). a: 100X. b: a higher (400X) magnification of a.

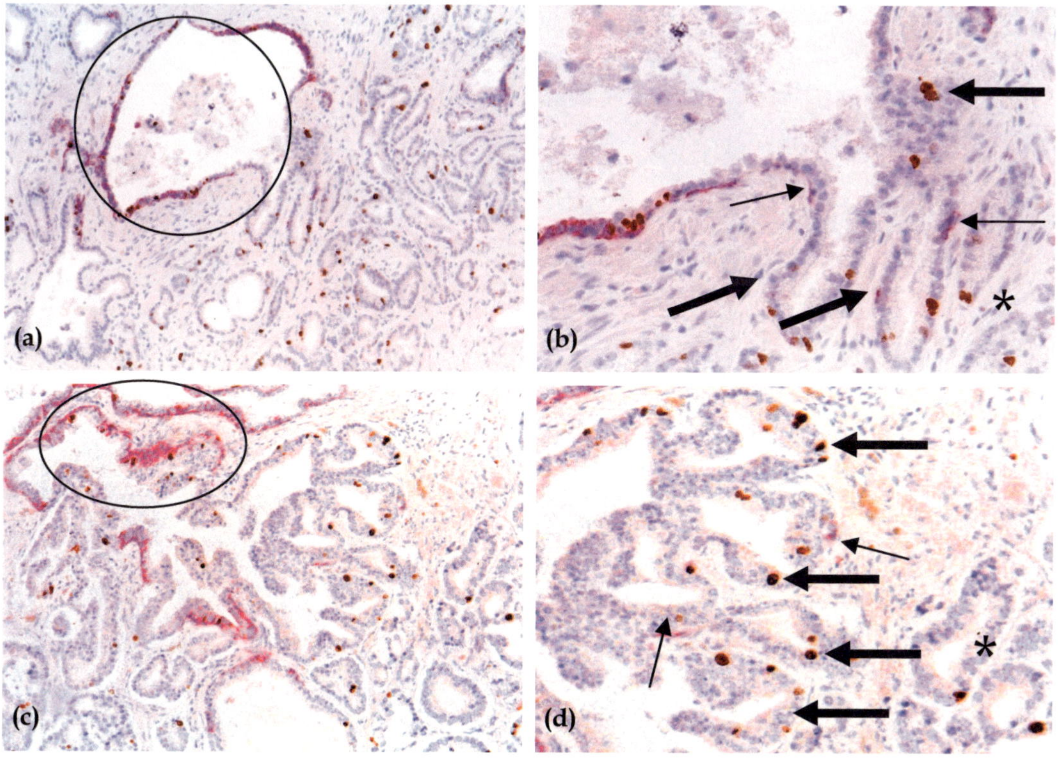

Fig. 12. Cell "budding" from normal epithelial structures. Double immunostained for CK34βE12 (red) and Ki-67 (brown). Circles identify normal epithelial structures. Thick arrows identify "budding" cell clusters. Thin arrows identify residual basal cells. Asterisks identify invasive cancers. a & c: 100X. b & d: a higher (400X) magnification of a and c, respectively.

D. Significantly higher expression of chromogranin A: In sections double immunostained for CK 34βE12 and chromogranin A, a neuroendocrine differentiation-related marker correlating with tumor progression and the status of hormone refractoriness [45-47], chromogranin A positive cells were exclusively or preferentially seen in epithelial structures with FBCLD (Fig 13). Compared to morphologically similar counterparts, microdissected epithelial structures with chromogranin A-positive cell clusters had a more than 5- and 7-fold lower expression of Micro-RNAs 146a and 146b-5p (miR-146a and miR-146b-5p; Fig 14), which have been documented to correlate with prostate tumor invasion and hormone refractoriness [38].

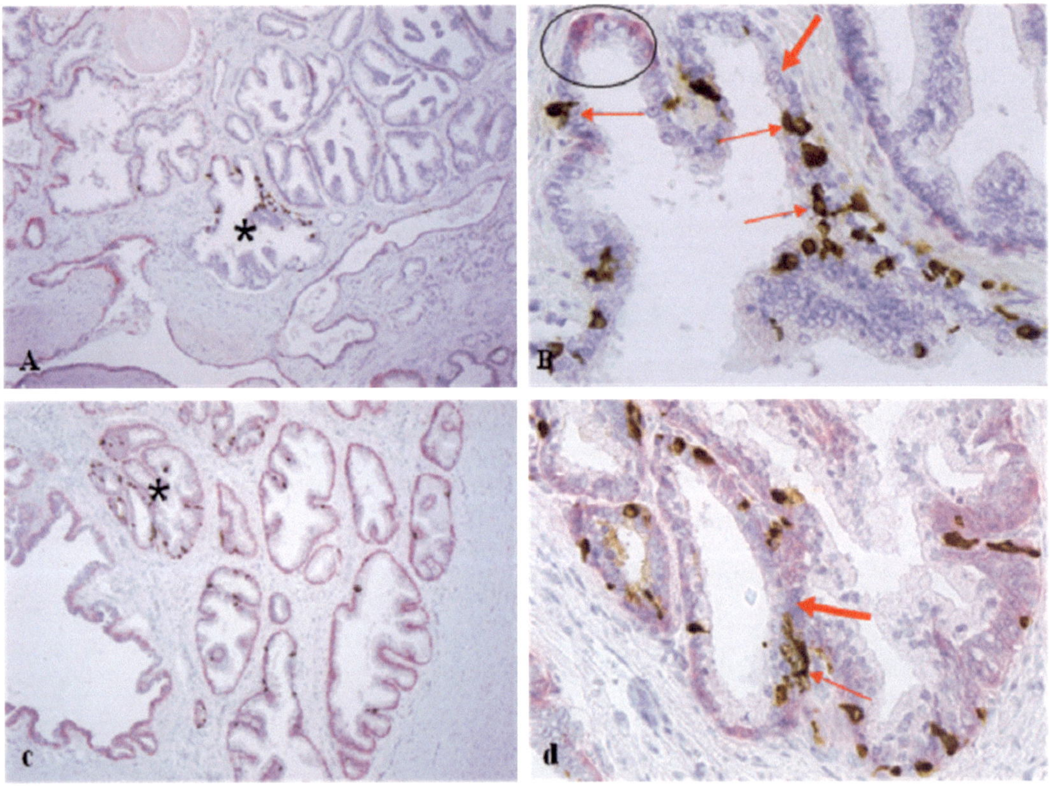

Fig. 13. Chromogranin A positive cells preferentially in epithelial structures with FBCLD. Double immunostained for CK βE12 (red) and chromogranin A (black). Thick arrows identify FBCLD. Thin arrows identify chromogranin A-positive cells. Circle identifies residual basal cells. Asterisks identify epithelial structures with FBCLD.

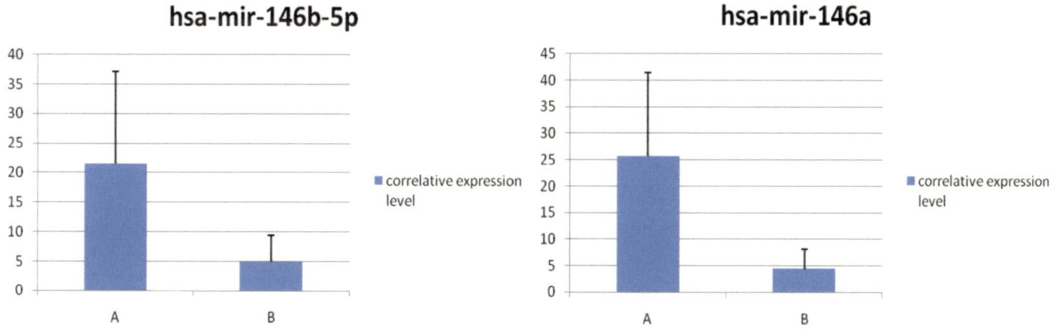

Fig. 14. Correlative expression levels of miR- 146a and 146b-5p in microdissected epithelial structures with (B) and without chromogranin-A positive cell clusters (A).

E. significantly elevated expression of tumor invasion-related genes: Compared to their adjacent counterpart associated with the residual basal cell layer within the same duct, microdissected cell clusters overlying FBCLD consistently had significantly higher expression of cell proliferation, apoptosis, angiogenesis, immuno-response, and stem cell related genes [38] (Fig 15; Table 6).

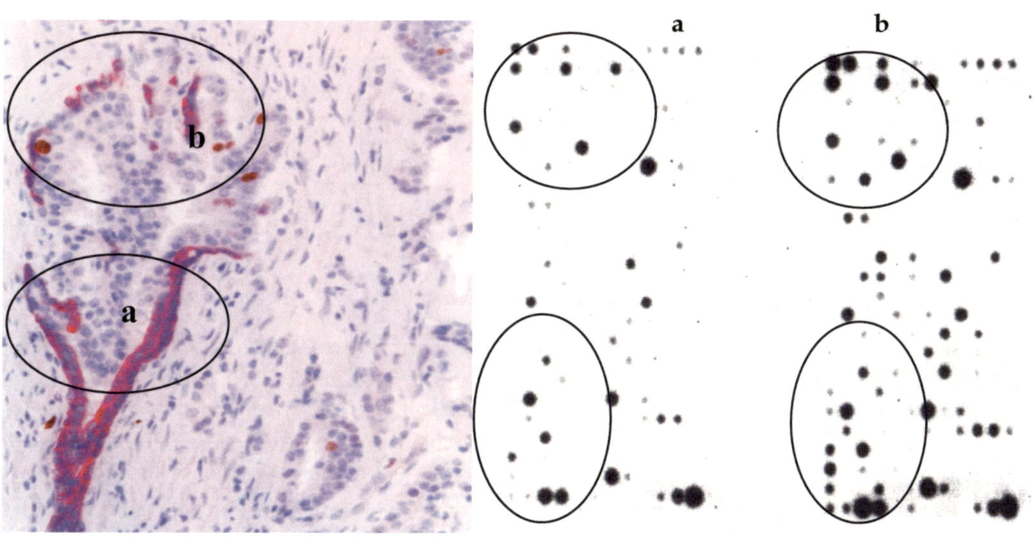

Fig. 15. Different gene expression profiles in cells overlying FBCLD and adjacent counterparts. Cells from these two locations were microdissected from frozen prostate sections, and subjected to RNA extraction, amplification, and gene expression profiling using our published protocols. Circles identify microdissected cells and differentially expressed genes.

#	Gene name	Potential functions	Fold changes
1	LIF	Growth factor	47.37
2	MCL1	Anti-apoptosis	6.72
3	TNFRSF7	Anti-apoptosis	7.91
4	KIT	Stem cell lineage marker	5.03
5	NCOR2	Stem cell lineage marker	5.45
6	ENG	Endothelial cell marker	6.38
7	ICAM2	Endothelial cell marker	12.12
8	KRT17	Epithelial cell marker	7.15
9	ITGA3	Cell-matrix adhesion	5.52
10	ITGB3	Cell-matrix adhesion	7.14
11	CCL2	Chemokine, cytokine, and receptor	14.33
12	CX3CL1	Chemokine, cytokine, and receptor	6.14
13	CCR1	Chemokine, cytokine, and receptor	5.19
14	CXCR4	Chemokine, cytokine, and receptor	12.81
15	TNFRSF10D	TNF receptor family	8.20
16	TNFRSF12A	TNF receptor family	5.35
17	TNFRSF25	TNF receptor family	8.52
18	TIMP1	ECM inhibitor	5.25
19	TIMP3	ECM inhibitor	7.87
20	MMP-26	Matrix metalloproteinase	-6.94
21	IL10	Interleukin and receptor	-9.50
22	IL12RB2	Interleukin and receptor	-7.02
23	IL6R	Interleukin and receptor	-7.24

Table 6. Differentially expressed genes between cells overlying FBCLD and their adjacent cells

The above alterations were consistently seen in all 17 cases with a high frequency of FBCLD, while were only seen in 1 (9.1%) of the 11 cases with a low frequency of FBCLD, and in none of the 22 cases with non-disrupted basal cell layers. Together, these findings suggest that the physical and functional status of the basal cell layer significantly impact the biological presentation of associated epithelial cells. These findings also suggest that malignant transformation and stromal invasion could occur in morphologically normal prostate tissues, and that FBCLD may represent a trigger factor for prostate tumor progression and invasion. To our best knowledge, our findings have not been previously reported by others. The most likely reasons are: [1] the enzyme theory has dominated the direction of researches in the field, and the roles of basal cells have been ignored, and [2] these alterations can be seen only by double immunohistochemistry to simultaneously elucidate the basal and epithelial cells. Double immunostaining, however, has not been commonly used in the clinical studies.

Our hypothesis of tumor invasion

Based on the above findings, we strongly believe that these normal appearing epithelial structures represent a population of maturation arrested tumor progenitors derived from monoclonal proliferation of genetically altered primitive stem cells at early stages of the prostate morphogenesis probably by trauma, radiation, inflammation, or other factors. These clusters retain the potential for unlimited cell proliferation or multi-lineage differentiation, and could progress directly to invasive lesions through two pathways: **(1) In situ malignant transformation, and (2) Progenitor-mediated cell budding.** These pathways are likely to contribute to early onset of prostate cancer at young ages, to biologically and clinically more aggressive prostate tumors, and also to highly heterogeneous genetic and biochemical profiles among prostate tumors.

The hypothesized main steps of tumor invasion

Our hypothesized main steps of invasion for these normal appearing epithelial structures are the followings:

1. At the early stage of prostate morphogenesis, the prostate of these patients exposed to external or internal insults, such as radiation, carcinogens, localized trauma, inflammation, or other factors, which caused permanent damages in the DNA structures of some primitive stem cells.
2. Localized DNA structural damages caused the inactivation of, or defects, in basal cell renewal-related genes, which impaired the basal cell replenishment process to replace the aged or injured basal cells, resulting in a "senesced" basal cell population with significantly reduced functions.
3. Localized DNA structural damages also caused the inactivation of, or defects in, apoptosis-, or cell cycle control related genes in the luminal cell population, which allow these cells to escape from programmed death, to continuously proliferate, and to generate their own vascular structures.
4. Deregulated proliferation in epithelial cells and impaired self-renewal in basal cells resulted in the overstretch and disassociation of the basal cell layer and the basement membrane, which lead to focal breakdown and degeneration of these two structures.
5. The degradation products of degenerated basal cells and the diffusible molecules of the overlying luminal cells function as self-epitopes to attract migration and infiltration of immunoreactive cells or auto-antibodies into the affected sites.
6. The direct physical contact between IRC and degenerated basal cells results in the discharge of the digestive enzymes from IRC, leading to the physical destruction of altered basal cell layers and the local basement membrane, resulting in a focal disruption in these structures.
7. As the epithelium is normally devoid of blood vessels and lymphatic ducts, and the basal cell layer is the sole source of several tumor suppressors, a FBCLD could lead to several focal alterations, including:
    a. A loss or reduction of tumor suppressors and the paracrine inhibitory functions, which allow the luminal cells to undergo elevated proliferation [48-52].
    b. Alterations in the permeability for oxygen or growth factors, which selectively triggers the exit of stem or progenitor cells from quiescence, and favor proliferation of cells overlying FBCLD [53-55].
    c. The exposure of luminal cells to different cytokines, which facilitates vasculogenic mimicry and tumor angiogenesis [56-57].

d. The physical contact between luminal and stromal cells augments the expression of stromal MMP, facilitating epithelial-mesenchymal transition (EMT) and cell motility [58-60].

e. The physical contact between luminal and immunoreactive cells directly cause genomic or cellular damages that trigger a cascade reaction of malignant transformation [61-64].

8. These alterations could individually or collectively trigger malignant transformation and stromal invasion through two different, but correlated pathways:

a. ***In situ* malignant transformation,** in which the entire basal cell layer undergoes extensive degeneration and multiple focal disruptions (Fig 16) that expose the entire luminal cell population directly to the stroma when all surrounding myoepithelial cells become degenerated. Although these cells might not possess all properties of invasive cancer cells, the changed microenvironment may act as a second "hit" to trigger a cascade reaction of malignant transformation that rapidly alters the genetic and biochemical profiles of these cells.

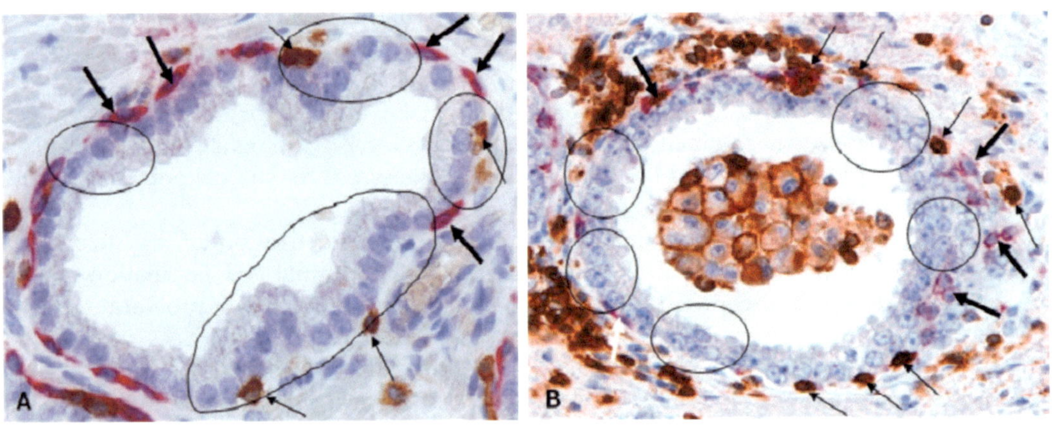

Fig. 16. Hypothesized model of *in situ* malignant transformation. Human prostate tissues double immunostained for CK34 βE12 (red) and LCA (brown). Circles identify FBCLD. Thick arrows identify residual basal cells. Thin arrows identify LCA-positive cells. Note that a vast majority of the epithelial cells are in direct physical contact with the stromal tissue. Also note that most LCA-positive cells are located at or near FBCLD. 300X.

b. **Progenitor-mediated cell budding,** in which focal basal cell degeneration-induced lymphocyte infiltration causes focal disruptions in the tumor capsules, which selectively favor proliferation and invasion of the overlying tumor stem cells or a biologically more aggressive cell clone. Cells overlying FBCLD gradually increases in volume and form finger-like projections invading into the surrounding stroma (Fig 17).

9. The above events may occur and progress immediately after the external or internal insults, leading to the onset of prostate cancer at young ages. On the other hand, cells of these normal appearing epithelial structures may become maturation-arrested after a few cycles of cells divisions, and remain idle until a new insult [65], representing "bad seeds for bad crops" at later ages.

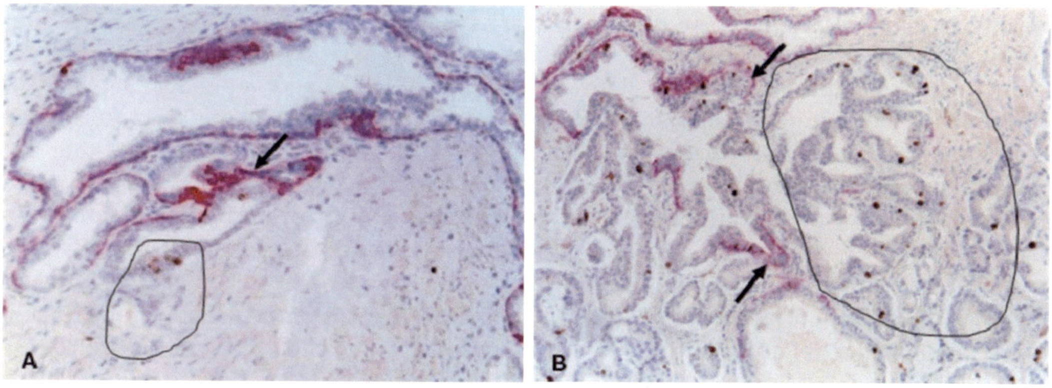

Fig. 17. Hypothesized model of progenitor-mediated cell budding. Human prostate tissues double immunostained for CK34 βE12 (red) and proliferation marker Ki-67 (brown). Thick arrows identify residual basal cell layers. Circles identify cell clusters budding from FBCLD. Note that cells budding from FBCLD are morphologically and immunohistochemically similar to adjacent invasive cancer cells, whereas they differ markedly from their adjacent counterpart within the same duct and associated with the residual basal cell layer. 200X.

The main differences between our hypothesis and other theories for tumor invasion

Based on our own and other findings, we had proposed that prostate tumor invasion is triggered by focal basal cell degeneration-induced aberrant infiltration of lymphocytes that causes focal disruptions in the tumor capsules, which selectively favor monoclonal proliferation and invasion of the overlying tumor stem or progenitor cells [38-39]. Our hypothesis differs from the enzyme theory of tumor invasion in five aspects: (1) the stage of tumor invasion, (2) the cellular origin of the invasive lesions, (3) the significance of the immunoreactive cells, (4) the significance of stromal cells, and (5) the potential approaches for interventions and prevention of tumor invasion. Our studies of breast tumors have obtained similar results and conclusions [66-74]. The new hypothesis presented in our current study is the expansion of our previous hypothesis with the following new points of views:

A. the preservation of large clusters of genetically damaged stem or progenitor cells: Our previous hypothesis proposes that cell clusters overlying FBCLD represent tumor stem or progenitor cells, which undergo a series of immunohistochemical and morphologic changes, and finally transform into invasive lesions [38]. Our current hypothesis suggests that it is also possible that multiple genetically damaged primitive stem or progenitor cells within the same site may generate large duct or acinar clusters that harbor the same genetic defects. These clusters may be formed immediately followed the external or internal insults during the early stage of morphogenesis, and progress rapidly, leading to the early onset of prostate cancer at young ages. These clusters could also become maturation arrested at patients' early ages, while they retain the potential for unlimited proliferation and multi- lineage differentiation, representing "bad seeds for bad crops" at later ages. Our speculation is supported by the results of our gene expression profiling studies, which have detected a over 5-fold higher expression of two stem cell lineage markers, KIT and NCOR2, in cell clusters overlying FBCLD compared to their adjacent counterpart associated with the residual basal cell layers [38] (Fig 15; Table 6).

B. direct transformation of the entire duct or acinar cluster into invasive lesions: Our previous hypothesis believes that invasive cells are derived exclusively or preferentially from monoclonal proliferation of stem or progenitor cells overlying FBCLD [38]. Our current hypothesis suggests that, in addition to monoclonal proliferation, it is possible that the entire duct or acinar cluster may directly transform into invasive lesions after the disappearance of all surrounding basal cells and the basement membrane.

C. angiogenesis by genetically altered tumor stem cells: Our previous hypothesis proposes that a subset of luminal cell clusters overlying FBCLD are in direct physical continuity with vascular- or lymphatic duct-like structures, which allows them to progress directly to metastasis [38]. Our current hypothesis further suggests that some normal appearing duct or acinar clusters may retain genetically damaged primitive stem cells that could manufacture their own blood vessels or lymphatic ducts, which directly lead to metastasis. Our speculation is consistently supported by our immunohistochemical findings, which show that some of the cell clusters overlying FBCLD appear to directly invade the vascular structures (Fig 11). Our speculation is also supported by the results of our gene expression profiling studies, which have detected a over 6- and 12-fold higher expression of two endothelial cell markers, END and ICAM2, respectively, in cell clusters overlying FBCLD compared to their adjacent counterpart associated with the residual basal cell layers [38] (Fig 15; Table 6).

D. Potential histological origin for cancer of unknown primary site: Cancer of unknown primary site (CUP) is one of the 10 most frequent cancers worldwide and ranks as the 4th most common cause of cancer-related death [22-24]. The development of early, uncommon, systemic metastasis, and resistance to therapy are hallmarks of this clinical entity. Currently, no consensus exists on whether CUP is a group of metastatic tumors with unidentified primaries or a distinct entity with unique genetic/phenotypic aberrations that define it as "primary metastatic disease [22-24]. The normal appearing epithelial structures seen in our current study may represent a potential histological origin for CUP for the following reasons: (1) they are morphologically indistinguishable from clear-cut normal prostate tissues under low magnification on H & E stained sections, which allow them to escape from early detection, (2) they retain the property of stem cells and appear to be able to directly invade the stroma and vascular structures, based on our previous [38] and current studies, and (3) they share the same DNA phenotype with invasive prostate cancer based on previous reports [14-17].

The significance of our hypothesis

During the past 30-years, the cancer research community has been predominantly, if not exclusively, focused on the roles of epithelial cells in prostate tumor progression and invasion. Hundreds and thousands of epithelium- derived molecules have been implicated in the development and progression of prostate cancers. However, only prostate-specific antigen (PSA) has been approved and validated as a clinical diagnostic marker and only growth factor- and androgen receptor-based therapeutic agents have been approved and validated for the clinical trials for prostate cancers. In addition, none of epithelium-derived markers has significant value in predicating the tumor biology or invasiveness, or in identifying the specific individuals with pending prostate cancer, or at higher risk to develop prostate cancer. These findings strongly suggest that the epithelium alone is very unlikely to be sufficient to trigger tumor progression and invasion.

Our hypothesis, if confirmed, could have several significant implications. Scientifically, it could lead to a new direction to explore novel approaches for early detection, intervention, and prevention of prostate tumor invasion. For example, as non-disrupted basal cell layers have significant inhibitory functions on epithelial cell growth, the development of therapeutic agents to stimulate basal cell growth or regeneration may provide a more effective approach for treatment and prevention of prostate cancer invasion. Clinically, it could potentially bring the following benefits:

1. Better recognition of these clusters may avoid misdiagnosis and facilitate early interventions, which may significantly improve prognosis.
2. Double immunohistochemical staining to assess the physical integrity of the basal cell layer, or an quantitative measurement of basal cell degeneration-related molecules in the blood or biopsies, may facilitate early identification of individuals at greater risk to develop invasive lesions.
3. As genetic alterations not only define the scope and extent of, but also precede, both biochemical and morphological alterations, elucidation of the genetic profile of these normal appearing duct or acinar clusters may lead to the identification of the specific molecules that trigger the initiation of prostate carcinogenesis, progression, and invasion.
4. Currently, the only established approach to monitor prostate tumor progression is repeat biopsy [28-31], which is costly and painful. Our technical approaches of assessing the physical and functional status of the basal cells may be used as a more reliable alternative for repeat biopsy to monitor tumor progression and invasion.

More importantly, our hypothesis may be also applicable to progression and invasion of other epithelium derived tumors.

2. Acknowledgment

This study was supported in part by grants DAMD17-01-1-0129, DAMD17-01-1-0130, and PC051308 from the US Congressionally Directed Medical Research Programs, grant BCTR0706983 from The Susan G. Komen Breast Cancer Foundation, grant 05AA from the AFIP/ARP joint research initiative project, grant 2008-02 from the US Military Cancer Institute and Henry Jackson Foundation, and grant 2006CB910505 from the Ministry of Chinese Science and Technology Department.

The tissue blocks or unstained tissue sections used in this study were obtained from our antibody testing service or collaborative research projects with the National Cancer Institute, Toms Jefferson University Medical School, Fairfax Hospital, Howard University Hospital, and Beijing 301 Hospital. The study was conducted in the Armed Forces Institute of Pathology with IRB approved protocols (05-AA and 07-DJ).

3. References

[1] Carruba G, Stefano R, Cocciaeliferro L. Intercellular communication and human prostate carcinogenesis. Ann NY Acad Sci. 2002; 963:156-68.

[2] Goldstein NS, Underhiel J, Roszka N, Neill JS. Cytokeratin 34 beta E-12 immunoreactivity in benign prostate acini. Quantitation, pattern assessment, and electron microscopic study. Am J Clin Pathol. 1999; 112:69-74.

[3] Bonkhoff H, Wernert N, Dhom G, Remberger K. Basement membranes in fetal, adult normal, hyperplastic and neoplastic human prostate. Virchows Arch A Pathol Anat Histopathol. 1991; 418:375-81.
[4] Kosir MA, Wang W, Zukowski KL, Tromp G. Degradation of basement membrane by prostate tumor heparanase. J Surg Res. 1999; 81:42-7.
[5] Bonkhoff H, Remberger K. Morphogenesis of benign prostatic hyperplasia and prostatic carcinoma. Pathology. 1998; 19:12-20.
[6] Bostwick DG. Prospective origins of prostate carcinoma. Prostate intraepithelial neoplasia and atypical adenomatous hyperplasia. Cancer. 1996;78: 330-6.
[7] Haggman MJ, Macoska JA, Wojno KJ, Oesterling JE. The relationship between prostate intraepithelial neoplasia and prostate cancer: critical issues. J Urol. 1997; 58:12-22.
[8] Bonkhoff H, Remberger K. Differentiation pathways and histogenetic aspects of normal and abnormal prostatic growth: a stem cell model. Prostate. 1996;28: 98-106.
[9] Barsky SH, Siegal GP, Jannotta F, Liotta LA. Loss of basement membrane components by invasive tumors but not by the benign counterparts. Lab Invest. 1983; 49:140-7.
[10] Goldfarb RH, Liotta LA. Proteolytic enzymes in cancer invasion and metastasis. Semin Thromb Hemost. 1986; 12: 294-307.
[11] Gardner WA, Culberson DE. Atrophy and proliferation in the young adult Prostate. J. Urol. 1987; 137(1): 53-6.
[12] Gardner WA. Hypothesis: Pediatric Origins of Prostate Cancer. Hum Path 1995; 26:1291-1292.
[13] Bennett BD, Gardner WA. Embryonal hyperplasia of the prostate. Prostate. 1985; 3 (7): 411-7.
[14] Malins DC, Polissar NL, Su Y, Gardner HS, Gunselman SJ. A new structural analysis of DNA using statistical models of infrared sepctra. Nat Med. 1997; 3: 927-30.
[15] Malins DC, Johnson PM, Barker EA, et al. Cancer-related changes in prostate DNA as men age and early identification of metastasis in prostate tumors. Proc Natl Acad Sci USA. 2003; 100: 5401-6.
[16] Malins DC, Anderson KM, Gilman NK, et al. Development of a cancer DNA phenotype prior to tumor formation. Proc Natl Acad Sci Sci USA. 2004; 101:10721-5.
[17] Malins DC, Gilman NK, Green VM, et al. A DNA phenotype in healthy prostates, conserved in tumors and adjacent normal cells, implies a relationship to carcinogenesis. Proc Natl Acad Sci USA. 2005; 102: 19093-6.
[18] Ashida S, Nakagawa H, Katagiri T, Furihata M, Liizumi M, Anazawa Y, et al. Molecular features of the transition from prostate intraepithelial neoplasia (PIN) to prostate cancer: genome-wide gene-expression profiles of prostate cancers and PINs. Cancer Res. 2004; 64:5963-72.
[19] Dawkins HJ, Sellner LN, Turbett GR, Thompson CA, Redmond SL, MeNeal JE, Cohen RJ. Distinction between intraductal carcinoma of the prostate (IDC-P), high-grade dysplasia (PIN), and invasive prostatic adecarcinoma, using molecular markers of cancer progression. Prostate. 2000; 44:265-70.
[20] Harvei S, Skijorten FJ, Robsahm TE, Berner A, Tretli S. Is prostaticibtraepithelial neoplasi in the transitio/central zone a true presursor of cancer? A long-tern retrospectivestudy in Norway. Br J Cancer. 1998; 78:46-9.

[21] Goeman L, Joniau S, Ponette D, Van der Aa F, Roskams T, Oyen R, Van Poppel H. Is low-grade prostatic intraepithelial neoplasia a risk factor for cancer. Prostate Cancer Prostatic Dis. 2003; 6:305-10.
[22] Pentheroudakis, G, Briasoulis, E, Pavlidis, N. Cancer of unknown primary site: missing primary or missing biology? Oncologist 2007; 12(4):418-425.
[23] Carlson HR. Carcinoma of unknown primary: searching for the origin of metastasis. JAAPA. 2009; 22(8): 18-21.
[24] Pentheroudakis, G, Pavlidis, N. Probing the unknown in cancer of unknown primary: which way is the right way? Ann Oncol. 2010, Jan 20 [Epub ahead of print].
[25] Parker SL, Tong T, Bolders S, Wingo PA. Cancer statistics. Cancer J Clin. 1997;47: 5-27.
[26] Bostwick DG. Prostatic intraepithelial neoplasia is a risk factor for cancer. Semin Urol Oncol. 1999; 17:187-9.
[27] Bostwick DG, Qian J, Frankel K. The incidence of high grade prostatic intraepithelial neoplasia in needle biopsies. J Urol. 1985; 154: 1791-4.
[28] Mostofi FK, Sesterhenn IA, Davis CJ Jr. Prostatic intraepithelial neoplasia (PIN): morphological clinical significance. Prostate Suppl. 1992; 4:71-7.
[29] Kasahara Y, Tsukada Y. New insights and future advances in cancer diagnostics: Limitations of conventional tumor markers. In: Nakarnura RM, Grody WW, Wu JT, Nagle RB, editors. Cancer Diagnostics: Current and future trends. Totowa, NJ: Humanna Press; 2004.
[30] Joniau S, Goeman L, Pennings J, Van Poppel H. Prostatic intraepithelial neoplasia (PIN): importance and clinical managment. Eur Urol. 2005; 48:379-85.
[31] Haggman MJ, Adolfsson J, Khoury S, Montie JE, Norlen J. Clinical managment of premalignant lesions of the prostate. WHO Collaborative Project and Consensus Conference on Public Health and Clinical Significance of Premalignant Alterations in the Genitourinary Tract. Scand J Urol Nephol Suppl. 2000; 205:44-9.
[32] Signoretti S, Waltregny D, Dilks J, et al. p63 is a prostate basal cell marker and is required for prostate development. Am J Pathol. 2000; 157:1769-75.
[33] Kurita T, Medina RT, Mills AA, Cunha GR. Role of p63 and basal cells in prostate. Development. 2004; 131: 4955-64.
[34] Zou Z, Zhang W, Young D, et al. Maspin expression profile in human prostate cancer (caP) and in vitro induction of maspin expression by androgen ablation. Clin Cancer Res. 2002; 8(5):1172-7.
[35] Cher ML, Biliran HR jr, Bhangat S, et al. Maspin expression inhibits osteolysis, tumor growth, and angiogenesis in animal model of prostate cancer bone metastasis. Proc Natl Acad Sci USA. 2003; 100(13):7847-52.
[36] Man YG, Shen T, Zhao YG, Sang QXA. Focal prostate basal cell layer disruptions and leukocyte infiltration are correlated events: A potential mechanism for basal cell layer degradations and tumor invasion. Cancer Detect Prev. 2005; 29:161-9.
[37] Man YG, Zhao CQ, Wang J, XL Chen. A subset of prostate basal cells lacks corresponding phenotypic markers. Pathology-Research & Practice. 2006; 202 (9): 651-62.
[38] Man YG, Gardner WA. Focal degeneration of basal cells and the resultant auto-immunoreactions: a novel mechanism for prostate tumor progression and invasion. Medical Hypoth. 2008; 70: 387-408.

[39] Man YG, Gardner WA. Bad seeds produce bad crops: a single step-process of prostate carcinogenesis and progression. Int J Biol Scien. 2008; 4: 246-58.
[40] Liu AJ, Wei LX, Gardner WA, Man YG. Correlated alterations in prostate basal cell layer and basement membrane. Int J Biol Sci. 2009; 5: 276-85.
[41] Man YG. A seemingly most effective target for early detection and intervention of prostate tumor Invasion. J Cancer. 2010; 1: 63-9.
[42] Man YG, Harley R, Mason J, Gardner WA. Contributions of leukocytes to tumor invasion and metastasis: the "piggy-back" hypothesis. Cancer Epidem 2010; 34(1): 3-6.
[43] Man YG, Mason J, Harley R, Kim YH, Zhu KM, Gardner WA. Leukocyte-facilitated tumor dissemination: a novel model for tumor cell dissociation and metastasis. J Cell Biochem. 2011 Feb 10. doi: 10.1002/jcb. 23035. [Epub ahead of print]
[44] Man YG, Fu SW, Liu AJ, Stojadinovic A, Izadjoo M, Chen L, Gardner WA. Aberrant expression of chromogranin A, miR-146a, and miR-146b-5p in prostate structures with focally disrupted basal cell layers: an early sign of invasion and hormone-refractory cancer? Submitted.
[45] Berruti A, Mosca A, Porpiglia F, Bollito E, Tucci M, Vana F, Cracco C, Torta M, Russo L, Cappia S, Saini A, Angeli A, Papotti M, Scarpa RM, Dogliotti L. Chromogranin A expression in patients with hormone negative prostate cancer predicts the development of hormone refractory disease. J Urol. 2007; 178(3 Pt1): 838-43.
[46] Grimaldi F, Valotto C, Barbina G, Visentini D, Trianni A, Cerruto MA, Zattoni F. The possible role of chromogranin A as a prognostic factor in organ-confined prostate cancer. Int J Biol Markers. 2006:21(4): 229-34.
[47] Berruti A, Mosca A, Tucci M, Terrone C, Torta M, Tarabuzzi R, Russo L, Cracco C, Bollito E, Scarpa RM, Angeli A, Dogliotti L. Independent prognostic role of circulating chromogranin A in prostate cancer patients with hormone-refractory disease. Endocr Relat Cancer. 2005; 12(1):109-17.
[48] Verona EV, Elkahloum AG, Yang J, Bandyopadhyay A, Yeh IT, Sun LZ. Transforming growth factor-beta signaling in prostate stromal cells supports prostate carcinoma growth by up-regulating stromal genes related to tissue remodeling. Cancer Res. 2007; 67(12):5737-46.
[49] Zhou W, Grandis JR, Wells A/ STAT3 is required but not sufficient for EGF receptor-mediated migration and invasion of human prostate carcinoma cell lines. Br J Cancer. 2006; 95(2):164-71.
[50] Chung IW, Baseman A, Assikis V, Zhau HE. Molecular insights into prostate cancer progression: the missing link of tumor microenvironment. J Urol. 2005;173(1):10-20.
[51] Boulikas T. Control of DNA replication by protein phosphorylation. Anticancer Res. 1994; 14: 2465-72.
[52] Boulikas T. Phosphorylation of transcription factors and control of the cell cycle. Crit Rev Eukaryot Gene Expr. 1995; 5: 1-77.
[53] Chakravarthy MV, Spangenhurg EE, Booth FW. Culture in low levels of oxygen enhances *in vitro* proliferation potential of satellite cells from old skeletal muscles. Cell Mol Life Sci. 2001; 58: 1150-8.
[54] Csete M, Walikonis J, Slawny N, et al. Oxygen-mediated regulation of skeletal muscle satellite cell proliferation and adipogrnesis in culture. J Cell Physical. 2001; 189:189-96.

[55] Studer L, Csete M, Lee SH. Enhanced proliferation, survival, and dopaminergic differentiation of CNS precursors in lowed pxygen. J Neurosci. 2000; 20: 7377-83.

[56] Klos KS, Wyszomierski SL, Sun M et al. c-erbB2 increases vascular endothelial growth factor protein synthesis via activation of mammalian target of rapamycin/p70S6K leading to increased angiogenesis and spontaneous metastasis of human breast cancer cells. Cancer Res. 2006; 66(4): 2028-37.

[57] Hendrix MJ, Seftor EA, Hess AR, Seftor RE. Vasculogenic mimicry and tumor-cell plasticity: lessons from melanoma. Nat Rev Cancer. 2003; 3(6): 411-21.

[58] Kang Y, Massague J. Epithelial-mesenchymal transition: twist in development and metastasis. Cell. 2004; 118: 277-9.

[59] Sato T, Sakai T, Noguchi Y, Takita M, Hirakawa S, Ito A. Tumor-stromal cell contact promotes invasion of human uterine cervical carcinoma cells by augmenting the expression and activation of stromal matrix metalloproteinases. Gynecol Oncol. 2004; 92: 47-56.

[60] Strizzi L, Bianco C, Normanno N. Epithelial mesenchymal transition is a characteristic of hyperplasias and tumors in mammary gland from MMTV-Criptol-1 transgenic mice. J Cell Physiol. 2004; 201:266-76.

[61] Smith, CJ, Gardner WA., Jr. Inflammation - Proliferation: Possible Relationships in the Prostate. In: D Coffey, N Bruchovsky, W Gardner, M Resnick, J Karr (Eds.) Current concepts in prostate cancer. Alan R. Liss, NY, NY 1987.

[62] Nelson G, Culberson DE, Gardner WA. Intraprostatic Spermatozoa. Hum Path. 1988; 19(1):119-20.

[63] Peek RM Jr, Mohla S, DuBois RN. Inflammation in the genesis and perpetuation of cancer: summary and recommendations from a national cancer institute-sponsored meeting. Cancer Res. 2005; 65: 8583-6.

[64] MacLennan GT, Eisenberg R, Fleshman RL et al. The influence of chronic inflammation in prostatic carcinogenesis: a 5-year follow-up study. J Urol. 2006; 176: 1012-6.

[65] Sell S, Pierce GB. Maturation arrest of stem cell differentiation is a common pathway for the cellular origin of teratocarcinomas and epithelial cancers. Lab Invest. 1994; 70, 6-22.

[66] Man YG, Tai L, Barner R, Vang R, Saenger JS, Shekitka KM, et al. Cell clusters overlying focally disrupted mammary myoepithelial cell layers and adjacent cells within the same duct display different immunohistochemical and genetic features: implications for tumor progression and invasion. Breast Cancer Res. 2003; 5: R231-41.

[67] Man YG, Sang QXA. The significance of focal myoepitehlial cell layer disruptions in breast tumor invasion: a paradigm shift from the "protease-centered" hypothesis. Exp Cell Res. 2004; 301: 103-18.

[68] Yousefi M, Mattu R, Gao C, Man YG. Mammary ducts with and without focal myoepithelial cell layer disruptions show a different frequency of white blood cell infiltration and growth pattern: Implications for tumor progression and invasion. AIMM. 2005; 13:30-7.

[69] Man YG, Zhang Y, Shen T, Vinh TN, Zeng X, Tauler J, Mulshine JL, Strauss BL. cDNA expression profiling identifies elevated expressions of tumor progression and invasion related genes in cell clusters of in situ breast tumors. Breast Cancer Res Treat. 2005; 89:199-208.

[70] Man YG, Nieburgs HE. A subset of cell clusters with malignant features in morphologically normal and hyperplastic breast tissues. Cancer Detect Prev. 2006; 30 (3):239-47.

[71] Man YG. Focal degeneration of aged or injured myoepithelial cells and the resultant auto-immunoreactions are trigger factors for breast tumor invasion. Medical Hypotheses. 2007; 69(6): 1340-57.

[72] Man YG. Bad seeds produce bad crops: a single-stage process of breast carcinogenesis. Bioscience Hypotheses. 2008; 1:147-155.

[73] Man YG. Tumor cell budding from focally disrupted tumor capsules: a common pathway for all breast cancer subtype derived invasion? Journal of Cancer 2010, 1: 27-31.

[74] Man YG, Grinkemeyer M, Izadjoo M, Stojadinovic A. Malignant transformation and stromal invasion from normal or hyperplastic tissues: true or false? J Cancer. 2011; 2: 386-400.

8

Strategies for Repeat Prostate Biopsies

Sisir Botta[1] and Martha K. Terris[2]
[1]*Chief of Urology, Augusta VA Medical Center*
[2]*Professor of Urology, Medical College of Georgia*
USA

1. Introduction

Despite urologists increasingly employing more extended prostate biopsy schemes for initial biopsies, the rate of repeat biopsies continues to rise [1]. Advances in technology and improved understanding of prostate cancer have not eliminated the questions surrounding the issue of repeat biopsies. What are the most reliable indications for repeat biopsy? How many biopsy cores should be obtained for optimal diagnostic yield to reduce the incidence of false-negative biopsies? What areas of the prostate should be biopsied to give the best diagnostic results? What is the best time interval between repeat biopsies? To how many repeat biopsy sessions should a patient be subjected?

Indications for repeat biopsy

Indications for repeat biopsies include sustained or worsening elevation of total serum PSA or other PSA parameters. Repeat biopsy has more recently been incorporated as part of active surveillance protocols to monitor patients with low-risk disease for reclassification to aggressive disease. The histology from the initial biopsy may also encourage repeat biopsy if high grade prostatic intraepithelial neoplasia (HGPIN) or atypical small acinar proliferation (ASAP) are identified. Risk factors such as family history of prostate cancer and African American race have not been evaluated as potential indications for repeat biopsy but often impact urologists attitudes toward encouraging patients to undergo repeat biopsy. Patient anxiety about the possibility of prostate cancer is another common but difficult to quantitate indication for repeat biopsy.

Prostate specific antigen as an indication for repeat biopsy

An elevated or rising PSA level is the most common indication for repeat prostate biopsies. A PSA level over 4.0ng/ml is generally accepted as an indication for initial biopsy while some urologists will biopsy for a PSA over 2.5ng/ml or adjust the acceptable upper limit of normal PSA for the patient's age. For repeat prostate biopsies after an initial set has been free of cancer, a PSA greater than 10.0ng/ml is agreed upon as a clear indication for the need for repeat biopsies while repeat biopsies are not felt to be strongly indicated for a PSA less than 4.0ng/ml [2-4]. PSA levels between 4.0 and 10.0 ng/ml present a significant range in which the indications for repeat biopsy are less obvious. Other PSA parameters can facilitate the decision to perform repeat biopsies. These include the percent-free PSA, PSA velocity (PSAV), PSA density (PSAD), and PSA density of the transition zone (PSAD-TZ).

Percent free PSA

The majority of serum PSA is attached either alpha1-antichymotrypsin or alpha2-macroglobulin. The remainder of the serum PSA that is not bound to these molecules is referred to as the "free" PSA and is decreased in the serum relative to the proportion of bound PSA in patients with cancer. The percentage of the total PSA (the bound and free PSA combined) that consists of the free PSA portion is termed the "percent free PSA." The percent free PSA has good utility in predicting cancer presence, specifically in men with PSA levels of 4 to 10 ng/ml. Catalona et al. demonstrated percent free PSA cutoff of less than 25% corresponded with the highest cancer detection rate and the least number of unnecessary biopsies [5]. Djavan et al. recommend a percent free PSA of less than 30% as one of the most accurate predictors of a positive repeat biopsy result [2]. Morgan et al. demonstrated that a percent free PSA less than 10% was a strong predictor for prostate cancer on repeat biopsy even after two negative prior biopsies with sensitivity and specificity of 91 and 86%, respectively [6]. Lee et al. report percent free PSA less than 10% yielded 90% and 91% specificity in the one repeat biopsy and greater than one repeat biopsy groups, respectively (57).

PSA density (PSAD)

PSAD is calculated by dividing the PSA value by the prostatic volume. This calculation targets the problem of PSA elevation caused by benign prostatic hyperplasia and, when elevated, has been shown to correlate with the existence of cancer. Keetch et al. evaluated density to assist in determining the need for a repeat biopsy [7]. Using a value of 0.15 ng/ml/cm3, they reported missing 35% of the cancers. However, in conjunction with a PSAV>0.75 ng/ml/yr, they had a detection rate of 46% on repeat biopsy, vs only 13% when both values were below the suggested cutoff. Djavan et al. evaluated PSAD, but showed increased utility when it was related to transition zone volume only, known as the PSA density of the transition zone (PSAD-TZ) [2]. Using a value of 0.13 and 0.26 ng/ml/cc for PSAD and PSA-TZ, respectively, they report sensitivities of 74 and 78% and specificities of 44 and 52%, respectively. Calculating the PSAD-TZ has the potential for a high rate of error due to the need for high resolution ultrasound equipment and an experienced sonographer since the margins of the transition zone are not as clearly demarcated as those of the entire prostate [3].

PSA velocity (PSAV)

PSAV is determined by taking the difference between two PSA values and dividing by the time interval between the two levels in years. PSAV has found more utility as a tool to predict recurrence in patients already diagnosed with prostate cancer but has been employed as a predictor of biopsy outcome as well. In a comparison to other PSA parameters, Borboroglu et al found that a PSAV of greater than 0.75 ng/ml/yr was the only statistically significant risk factor for prostate cancer detection on biopsy [8]. However, the European Randomized Study of Screening for Prostate Cancer failed to show clinical utility for either PSA velocity or PSA doubling time [9]. Vickers et al. reported that prostate specific antigen velocity was statistically associated with cancer risk but had low predictive accuracy (AUC 0.55, $p<0.001$) (55). PSA doubling time (PSADT) is another measure of PSA change over time but has similarly demonstrated more utility in the prediction of prostate cancer aggressiveness than as an indication for repeat biopsy.

Many investigators have now come to the conclusion that no single PSA parameter is adequate to indicate the need for repeat biopsies. Keetch et al. determined that using only

PSAV greater than 0.75 ng/ml/yr would miss a large number of cancers and recommended combining the PSAV other parameters [7]. Djavan et al. recommend the combination of a percent free PSA of less than 30% and/or a PSAD-TZ greater than or equal to 0.26 ng/ml/cc as the most accurate predictor of a positive repeat biopsy result in patients with PSA levels between 4 and 10 ng/ml [2]. Busby and Evans recommend a combination of total PSA, percent free PSA, PSAD, and PSAV based on analysis of the published data on each of these parameters [3]. Their recommended PSA-based indications for repeat biopsy include any patient with a PSA in the 4-10 ng/ml range and a percent free PSA less than 25%. For patients with a PSA between 4-10ng/ml and percent free greater than 25%, repeat biopsies are recommended if they have a PSAD greater than 0.15ng/ml/cc and a PSAV greater than 0.75 ng/ml/yr, or a PSAV greater than 1 ng/ml/yr, or a PSAD-TZ greater than 0.26 ng/ml/yr. Both Djavan et al. and Busby and Evans recommend repeat biopsy in any patient with a PSA greater than 10 ng/ml, regardless of the other parameters. Busby and Evans qualify this recommendation by stating patients with PSA >10 ng/ml with inflammation noted histologically should have a trial of antibiotics and repeat PSA before considering repeat biopsy.

Repeat biopsy for active surveillance protocols

As PSA-based prostate cancer screening has expanded, some have noted the overdetection of cancer that would not have been detected in the absence of screening programs (51). The risks and benefits of invasive therapy for prostate cancer have been debated. Active surveillance (AS) has become established for low-risk patients to offset or delay the risks of invasive therapy. AS regimens monitor these low-risk patients via repeat prostate biopsies at fixed intervals to assess for those candidates with disease progression who should be offered radical treatment. The optimal parameters for timing of repeat prostate biopsy have not been definitively established (52). The European Randomised Study of Screening for Prostate Cancer (ERSPC) has instigated a prospective observational study, the Prostate Cancer Research International: Active Surveillance (PRIAS). This protocol includes a schedule for follow-up of low-risk prostate cancer patients that begins with a first repeat biopsy at 1 year after diagnosis. Bul et al. report that 21.5% of patients were reclassificatied to higher risk. This reclassification was significantly influenced by the number of initial positive cores, higher PSA density, and PSA doubling time (PSA-DT) < 3years (52).

Van den Bergh et al. reports that PSAV and PSA-DT carry sparse evidence for their role as prognisticators, especially in active surveillance (53). They report some consensus of the unfavorable prognosis of PSA-DT < 3years and the favorable prognosis of PSA-DT > 10 years or decreasing PSA level (53). The best method of calculation, number of measurements, and time interval of measurements remains unknown.

Repeat biopsy for high grade prostatic intraepithelial neoplasia

High Grade Prostatic Intraepithelial Neoplasia (HGPIN) is characterized by prostatic glands in which the epithelial cells exhibit the nuclear enlargement and prominent nucleoli characteristic of prostatic adenocarcinoma, yet with a preserved basal cell layer. While the presence of a basal cell layer excludes the diagnosis of invasive cancer, HGPIN is thought to be a precursor to invasive adenocarcinoma [10]. Evaluating pathology trends on 62,537 initial prostate needle core biopsies submitted by office-based urologists, processed at a single pathology laboratory, isolated high grade PIN was diagnosed in 4.1% of the biopsies

[11]. In a referral academic practice employing extended field biopsies for initial prostate tissue sampling, 22% of cases exhibited isolated HGPIN [12].

After sextant biopsies showing HGPIN, 80% of patients demonstrated cancer on repeat biopsy [13]. With extended biopsy schemes showing HGPIN, the rate of cancer detection on repeat biopsies was only 23% [14]. This decreased cancer detection rate after extended biopsy schemes is probably due to the better sampling and increased likelihood of identifying co-existing cancer and HGPIN on the initial extended biopsy procedure.

Low grade prostatic intraepithelial neoplasia does not carry the same risk of concomitant cancer. Zlotta et al. found that low grade PIN was associated with subsequent cancer on repeat biopsies in 10.7% of patients with a PSA was between 4 and 10ng/ml and in none of the cases when PSA was ≤4ng/ml [15]. Low grade PIN is not considered an indication for repeat biopsy unless other factors such as an elevated PSA increase the suspicion of prostate cancer. In fact, the notation of the presence of low grade PIN has been discouraged from being mentioned in pathology reports.

Most experts strongly recommend repeat biopsy for any patient with HGPIN on initial biopsy [3,16]. If HGPIN is again identified on repeat biopsy but no cancer diagnosed, follow-up PSA and examination in 6 months is recommended.

Repeat biopsy for atypical small acinar proliferation

Atypical Small Acinar Proliferation (ASAP) is a focus of small glands that have the cytologic appearance of malignancy; however, the presence or absence of the basal cell layer is equivocal [17]. Rather than a pre-malignant lesion, this finding is felt to often represent invasive cancer that is simply difficult for the pathologist to clearly identify due to issues such the plane of sectioning. In patients with ASAP, cancer found on repeat biopsy is most likely to be in the same region of the prostate as was the ASAP. Repeat biopsy samples in patients with ASAP are found to have cancer in approximately 40–50% of cases [13]. Zhou et al. affirmed these findings with the report that of patients diagnosed with ASAP, 51.0% were diagnosed with prostate cancer on repeat biopsy (56). This rate has not changed in the era of extended biopsy schemes.

ASAP is considered an absolute indication for repeat biopsy [3,16]. Negative repeat biopsies require close follow-up.

Impact of prostate volume on repeat biopsies

Prostate volume is an important parameter when deciding whether or not to perform a repeat biopsy. Rietbergen et al. found that the most important factor responsible for failure to diagnose these cancers at the primary screening was a large prostate volume in the European Randomized Study for Screening for Prostate Cancer [18]. One explanation is the possibility that these patients' increased PSA levels are primarily due to the volume of prostatic hyperplasia. The lower biopsy yield in larger prostates has also been attributed to undersampling since a proportionally smaller amount of tissue is sampled relative to the total prostate volume. The potential for undersampling in large prostates is compounded by the fact that larger glands tend to harbor smaller volume tumors [19].

Remzi et al. showed that there were increased numbers of cancers discovered on repeat biopsy for those with prostate volume 20-80 cc and for those whose TZ volume was 9-40 cc [20]. Beyond these size limits, they discourage repeat biopsy unless there is very strong suspicion of cancer based on other characteristics. Basillote et al. also demonstrated increased false-negative rates in patients with increased prostate volumes [21]. Using extended biopsy schemes for initial biopsies, Ung et al. found no increased prostate cancer detection rates in larger volume prostates [22]. However, Sajadi et al found a much lower cancer detection rate with repeat "saturation" biopsies in large prostates compared to smaller glands (57% positive biopsy rate in glands less than 37cc and only 7% for larger glands) [23].

In practical terms, large prostates can often result in an initial biopsy that shows no malignancy. At least one set of repeat, extended biopsy of moderately enlarged prostates in patients with persistent concern about cancer appear justified. For extremely enlarged prostates (over 80 cc) the utility of repeat biopsies is unclear.

Repeat biopsies and inflammation

Prostatic inflammation often causes an increase in serum PSA levels. While the pathogenesis of inflammation-related PSA elevation is not completely understood, it is theorized to result from either leakage of PSA from epithelial cells into the serum or through stimulation of PSA production by epithelial cells through inflammatory-mediated substances [24, 25]. Nadler et al. noted that prostate inflammation and volume were the most important factors resulting in PSA elevations in those without prostate cancer [26]. Okada et al. found that histologically evident acute inflammation was the only independent determinant of serum PSA in those with prostates smaller than 25 cc [24]. While inflammation may inflate total PSA, it does not appear to influence the percent-free PSA [27]. To further complicate matters, we have demonstrated that the histologic finding of inflammation increases with sequential repeat biopsies [1]. Abouassaly et al have shown that the presence of inflammation can increase likelihood of the histologic diagnosis of ASAP, creating another avenue by which inflammation can stimulate the performance of unnecessary repeat biopsies [28]. Although it has not been clinically validated, interval antibiotic administration to correct PSA elevation secondary to histologic inflammation may help PSA reach its true baseline [3].

Time interval to repeat biopsies

Patients at high risk for existing cancer should undergo repeat biopsy without delay, recommendations vary between 2 and 6 weeks [2, 3]. High risk patients include those with ASAP or HGPIN. Others fitting this high-risk category include patients without inflammation on initial biopsy whose PSA is >10 ng/ml or with both a PSA between 4 and 10 ng/ml and percent free <10%. Other risk factors such as family history of prostate cancer and African American race have not been studied in relationship to the interval between initial and repeat prostate biopsies.

For patients who are not at high risk, a repeat PSA in 3 to 6 months to allow for calculation of PSAV has been recommended. While many patients will be relieved to postpone repeat biopsy for a few months, many will find the wait very anxiety-provoking. There is certainly no contraindication to more expeditious repeat biopsy in a very anxious patient.

Patient preparation

Patient preparation for repeat biopsies is a duplicate of the preparation used for initial biopsy in many facilities. Most urologists have the patient give themselves an enema before the procedure [29]. While taking aspirin or non-steroidal anti-inflammatory drugs is not an absolute contraindication to prostate biopsy, avoiding these medications for at least 10 days prior to the procedure is preferable. Some of the more aggressive extended biopsy schemes are performed under general anesthesia or with monitored sedation. Without the systemic control of discomfort, periprostatic injection of local anesthetic is strongly recommended before subjecting an patient to extended biopsy schemes [30].

A short course of an oral fluoroquinolone antibiotic is the most common preparation [29]. Since these patients have already had a course of antibiotics for their prior biopsy and may have taken an even longer course of antibiotics if treated for prostatic inflammation, the possibility of resistant bacteria should be considered [31]. Pre-procedure urine culture, extended oral antibiotic coverage, or additional prophylaxis with an intravenous or intramuscular injection of an aminoglycoside should be considered.

Location and number of repeat biopsy cores

Hong et al. demonstrated that prostate cancer detection rates on repeat biopsy vary as a function of the extent of the initial biopsy [32]. If the prior negative biopsy was a sextant scheme, the cancer detection rate was 39% with a repeat extended biopsy, whereas if the prior negative biopsy was an extended scheme, the cancer detection rate was 28%. In general, areas not sampled on initial biopsy have higher rates of cancer detection when those areas were sampled on repeat biopsies. Therefore, repeat biopsy schemes typically consist of extended biopsy schemes designed to sample the areas of the prostate incompletely sampled by the initial biopsy. Repeat biopsy techniques also target those anatomic areas of the prostate where malignancy is more likely to reside. Repeat extended biopsy schemes consist of the classic sextant biopsy pattern plus various combinations of anteriorly directed biopsies that are designed to sample the transition zone, posterolateral sampling which includes the anterior horn of the peripheral zone, and anterior apical biopsies.

Directed biopsies

Directed biopsies were the initial approached used in conjunction with prostate ultrasound for prostatic sampling. With this approach, biopsies are taken only from areas that were suspicious on the ultrasound images and/or digital rectal examination. This method was far superior to the previously utilized digitally directed "blind" biopsies, however, with the current predominance of non-palpable isoechoic prostate tumors, biopsy sites limited to either sonographically hypoechoic lesions or areas of palpable abnormality have limited utility [1]. Most current extended biopsy schemes include any region in which an abnormality-directed biopsy would sample but an occasional directed biopsy in conjunction with the performance of an extended biopsy scheme may be useful in selected patients. . In addition, patients with ASAP should have additional cores obtained from the region of the ASAP [14]. This is in contrast to patients who are found to have HGPIN, where the finding of cancer on repeat biopsy is equally likely throughout the gland [14]. Some investigators have found a slight increase in cancer detection rates on repeat biopsies in the area from which the original biopsy containing HGPIN was taken [33,34]. These authors recommend that additional biopsies should be performed in the area previously harboring HGPIN.

Sextant biopsies

The sextant biopsy scheme, a method of obtaining spatially separated biopsies from each sextant of the prostate, was designed to improve the odds of sampling clinically inapparent tumors. These biopsy sites were originally described in mid-lobe parasagittal plane at the apex, mid-gland and base bilaterally. Although far superior to directed biopsies, sextant biopsies maintain a false negative rate between 15% and 34% based on repeated biopsies and computer simulations [1]. While sufficient for histologic confirmation of the presence of cancer in patients with very abnormal digital rectal examinations and elevated PSA levels, use of sextant biopsies alone is generally considered inadequate for routine initial or repeat biopsies [2,3,16]. "Extended" biopsy is the terminology typically used to refer to greater than six biopsy cores taken in the sextant fashion. Despite falling out of favor as the sole approach to prostate sampling, sextant biopsies in conjunction with additional biopsies as part of an extended biopsy scheme continue to contribute significantly to the successful detection of prostate cancer [35].

Lateral biopsies

Pathologic analysis of radical prostatectomy specimens suggests that small prostate cancers occur in the posterolateral portion of the gland. These cancers are still in the peripheral zone where most prostate cancers reside, but are in the portion of the transition zone that wraps anteriorly and laterally. This area is occasionally termed the "anterior horn" in the literature. Stamey initially described the concept of targeting this area of the prostate with laterally placed sextant biopsies [36]. Eskew et al. introduced the first extended biopsy scheme for routine cancer detection and included the use of lateral biopsies [37]. The 5 regions included the standard sextant biopsies in the mid-lobe parasaggital plane bilaterally as well as two biopsies from lateral aspect of the prostate and three biopsies from the midline. Of the 119 patients studied, 48 (40%) were found to have prostate cancer on the biopsy, of which 17 (35% of cancers identified) were only detected in the additional non-sextant sites. Through analysis of the cancer detection yield of each individual biopsy site, Presti et al. first popularized the 10-core biopsy scheme combining routine mid-lobar sextant biopsies plus lateral biopsies on each side for routine use in all patients [38]. This technique perfected the concept of extended biopsies proposed by Eskew et al by determining the number and location of biopsies that resulted in the maximum cancer detection rate for the minimum number of biopsies performed. Lateral biopsies of the peripheral zone at the base and mid gland were added to the routine sextant biopsy regimen for a total of 10 systematic biopsies of the peripheral zone. Mian et al. utilized a 10-biopsy schema including the six sextant biopsies and two biopsies from each of the anterior horns of the peripheral zone [39]. This resulted in cancer detection in 33% of initial biopsies in 939 men. Babaian et al first introduced the use of extended biopsy schemes for repeat biopsies in 278 patients with prior negative prostate biopsies [40]. This 11-core strategy included sextant, lateral and anterior transition zone biopsies bilaterally.

Transition zone biopsies

We initially introduced the biopsy technique to sample the anterior prostate, or transition zone, in order to evaluate patients with cancer diagnosed by transurethral resection of the prostate (TURP) for residual/recurrent disease [41]. Anterior biopsies detected residual cancer in 47% of patients in whom cancer was detected by TURP. While routine performance of anterior biopsies was shown to be not warranted, anterior biopsies have been recommended as part of repeat extended field biopsies [32]. Liu et al. evaluated 116 patients who underwent sextant plus transition zone biopsies after prior negative sextant biopsies [42]. Overall, 36 (31.0%) were found to have prostate cancer while 11 (9.5%) demonstrated cancer only in the transition zone. Most investigators suggest 2 cores bilaterally from the transition zone while others recommend 3 biopsies from each side of the prostate in an anterior version of the sextant biopsy scheme [32, 39]. Adjusting the number of anterior biopsies according to the size of the transition zone, spacing them approximately 1cm apart, has also been suggested [43].

Transition zone biopsies should be performed near the midline, as close as possible to the urethra and anterior fibromuscular stroma. Transition zone biopsies are taken by advancing the biopsy needle through the posterior capsule of the prostate, into the peripheral zone to within 2-3 mm of the sonographically evident surgical capsule between the transition zone and the peripheral zone before firing; in prostates that extend far anteriorly (determined by the anteroposterior dimension of the transition zone exceeding 2cm), the needle is advanced through the surgical capsule and into the transition zone in order to sample the anterior-most tissue where transition zone tumors most frequently reside [41].

Midline biopsies

Performance of biopsies in the midline of the prostate has been utilized by some authors [37]. These biopsies have a very low yield compared to sextant, anterior, or lateral biopsies and have not been widely accepted by other investigators [38]. Even proponents of routinely performed extended field biopsies, find that these midline cores provide the least additional information [39,40].

Anterior apical biopsies

The entire apex of the prostate is composed of peripheral zone where it wraps around the caudal extent of the transition zone Although extended biopsy schemes sample the posterior and lateral apex, the anterior apex of the prostate is potentially undersampled. Several investigators have independently recommended that additional cores should be taken from the anterior apex on repeat biopsy [16, 44, 45].

Saturation biopsies

One of the most aggressive biopsy approaches suggested in patients with prior negative biopsies is the "saturation biopsy" technique [46]. The approach was originally described as multiple cores take from each of the 12 midlobe and lateral sextant locations as well as the transition zone. A mean of 23 cores were performed under anesthesia as an outpatient procedure. Subsequent use of a 24-core office-based saturation biopsy approach was described by Jones et al [47]. The utility of saturation biopsies for initial biopsies has been shown to be limited but use as a repeat biopsy scheme, with or without anesthesia may have a role in some patients [23, 48]. In patients who did not tolerate their initial biopsies without anesthesia very well, proceeding with performance of saturation biopsy under anesthesia rather than repeat, less extensive biopsies without anesthesia is often the more humane option.

Transperineal template biopsies

Igel et al. advocate employing the transperineal template apparatus used for brachytherapy seed implants for extensive repeat biopsy sampling [49]. In there follow-up study in which over 80% of patients had had at least 2 prior transrectal biopsy procedures, cancer was detected in 37% of patients [50]. The method seems to be superior in sampling the transition zone as 77% of the cancers in these patients with prior negative transrectal biopsies had cancer in the transition zone biopsies. Some experts question the accuracy of the assumed location of biopsy placement by this method [16].

How many repeat biopsy sessions is enough?

Unfortunately, negative repeat biopsies do not often settle the question of the presence or absence of prostate cancer. Multiple repeat biopsy procedures that reveal no cancer despite a rising PSA cause increasing frustration for the patient and urologist, alike. In men with serum PSA levels between 4 and 10ng/ml, the European Randomized Study for Screening for Prostate Cancer demonstrated cancer detection rates on biopsies 1, 2, 3 and 4 of 22% (231 out of 1051), 10% (83 of 820), 5% (36 of 737) and 4% (4 out of 94), respectively [2]. The pathological and biochemical features of cancers detected on the first two sets of biopsies were similar but cancers detected on the third and fourth sets had lower grade, stage and volume. Even before the widespread use of extended biopsy protocols, a significant decreased yield after the third set of biopsies was demonstrated [1]. Therefore, after 2 or 3 sets of negative biopsies, further repeat biopsies appeared to be justified in very young, healthy patients where there is a very high suspicion of cancer despite two sets of negative findings [2]. Resnick et al. noted the risk of clinically insignificant disease in those patients diagnosed with prostate cancer on first repeat biopsy, on second repeat biopsy, and on third repeat biopsy of 31.1%, 43.8%, and 46.8%, respectively ($p<0.01$) (54). Conversely, the risk of adverse pathology in the above groups was determined to be 64.6%, 53.0%, and 52.0%, respectively ($p<0.01$) (54).

Complications of repeat prostate biopsy

Prostate biopsy is not entirely free from morbidity, especially in the setting of serial biopsies. In a cohort of greater than 75,000 patients, Nam et al. reported that the risk of post-biopsy hospital admission rates have increased from 1.0% in 1996 to 4.1% in 2005. There is concern for fluoroquinolone resistant infections, and the AUA Best practices statement recommends antibiotic prophylaxis.

In the prospective European Prostate Cancer Detection Study, Djavan et al. report minor or no discomfort was observed in 92% and 89% of patients at first and re-biopsy, respectively (p _ 0.29). Immediate morbidity was minor and included rectal bleeding (2.1% versus 2.4%, p _ 0.13), mild hematuria (62% versus 57%, p _ 0.06), severe hematuria (0.7% versus 0.5%, p _ 0.09) and moderate to severe vasovagal episodes (2.8% versus 1.4%, respectively, p _ 0.03). Delayed morbidity of first and re-biopsy was comprised of fever (2.9% versus 2.3%, p _ 0.08), hematospermia (9.8% versus 10.2%, p _ 0.1), recurrent mild hematuria (15.9% versus 16.6%, p _ 0.06), persistent dysuria (7.2% versus 6.8%, p 0.12) and urinary tract infection (10.9% versus 11.3%, respectively, p _ 0.07). Major complications were rare and included urosepsis (0.1% versus 0%) and rectal bleeding that required intervention (0% versus 0.1%, respectively) (59). Hence, repeat biopsy was recommend repeat after 6 weeks with no significant difference in pain or morbidity.

2. Conclusions

The primary indications for repeat biopsies are a persistently elevated/rising PSA , active surveillance protocols, or suspicious histology on initial biopsies. Variations of PSA measurement may help determine the need for repeat biopsies. Repeat biopsies should include a minimum of 14 cores including parasagittal and lateral sextant biopsies and 2 additional cores obtained from the right and left anterior apex. For patients in whom repeat biopsies fail to identify cancer despite a high clinical suspicion, consideration for repeat 14-core biopsy with additional 4 to 6 transition zone biopsies or a saturation biopsy approach seems warranted. Repeat biopsies after 2 or 3 biopsies fail to reveal cancer have limited yield. There is no significant increase in morbidity for repeat biopsy procedures after six weeks.

Further areas of study include determining any difference in the indications for repeat biopsy in patients with risk factors such as a family history of prostate cancer or African

American patients. Artificial neural networks incorporating the multiple potential indicators of repeat biopsies have yet gain the ease of use necessary for routine clinical care but may have future utility. Advanced sonographic technological such as power Doppler and elastography as well as biopsy needles that provide feedback on tissue characteristics have shown some promise. Additionally, transrectal MRI-guidance or MR spectroscopy for prostate biopsy have also been performed with promising results. Adjustment of biopsy schemes to allow tailoring to individual patient prostate size and shape may also improve yield without continued increase in the total number of biopsies performed

3. References

Papers of particular interest, published recently,have been highlighted as:
• Of importance
• • Of major importance

[1] •Terris MK. Prostate biopsy strategies: past, present, and future. Urol Clin North Am. 2002, 29: 205-212. A historical review of the development of prostate biopsies.

[2] ••Djavan B, Remzi M, Schulman CC, Marberger M, Zlotta AR: Repeat prostate biopsy: who, how and when? A review. Eur Urol. 2002, 42:93-103. Summary of the results of multiple publications from the European Prostate Cancer Detection study to clinically useful recommendations.

[3] •Busby JE, Evans CP: Determining variables for repeat prostate biopsy. Prostate Cancer Prostatic Dis. 2004, 7: 93-98. An integrative approach to utilizing the factors utilized for determining the need for repeat biopsies.

[4] Djavan B, Fong YK, Ravery V, Remzi M, Horninger W, Susani M, Kreuzer S, Boccon-Gibod L, Bartsch G, Marberger M. Are repeat biopsies required in men with PSA levels < or =4 ng/ml? A Multiinstitutional Prospective European Study. Eur Urol. 2005, 47:38-44

[5] Catalona WJ, Partin AW, Slawin KM, et al.: Use of the percentage of free prostate-specific antigen to enhance differentiation of prostate cancer from benign prostatic disease: a prospective multicenter clinical trial. JAMA 1998, 279:1542-1547.

[6] Morgan TO, McLeod DG, Leifer ES, Murphy GP, Moul JW: Prospective use of free prostate-specific antigen to avoid repeat prostate biopsies in men with elevated total prostate-specific antigen. Urology. 1996, 48: 76-80.

[7] Keetch DW, McMurtry JM, Smith DS, Andriole GL, Catalona WJ: Prostate specific antigen density versus prostate specific antigen slope as predictors of prostate cancer in men with initially negative prostatic biopsies. J Urol 1996; 156 : 428–431.

[8] Borboroglu PG, Comer SW, Riffenburgh RH, Amling CL: Extensive repeat transrectal ultrasound guided prostate biopsy in patients with previous benign sextant biopsies. J Urol 2000, 163: 158–162.

[9] Raaijmakers R, Wildhagen M, Ito K: Prostate-Specific Antigen change in the European Randomized Study of Screening for Prostate Cancer, section Rotterdam. Urology. 2004, 63: 316–320.

[10] Häussler O, Epstein JI, Amin MB, Heitz PU, Hailemariam S: Cell proliferation, apoptosis, oncogene, and tumor suppressor gene status in adenosis with comparison to benign prostatic hyperplasia, prostatic intraepithelial neoplasia, and cancer. Hum Pathol. 1999, 30:1077-1086.

[11] Orozco R, O'Dowd G, Kunnel B, Miller MC, Veltri RW: Observations on pathology trends in 62,537 prostate biopsies obtained from urology private practices in the United States. Urology. 1998, 51:186–195.
[12] Schoenfield L, Jones JS, Zippe CD, et al.: The incidence of high-grade prostatic intraepithelial neoplasia and atypical glands suspicious for carcinoma on first-time saturation needle biopsy, and the subsequent risk of cancer. BJU Int. 2007, 99: 770-774.
[13] Meng MV, Shinohara K, Grossfeld GD: Significance of high-grade prostatic intraepithelial neoplasia on prostate biopsy. Urol Oncol 2003, 21: 145–151.
[14] O'Dowd GJ, Miller MC, Orozco R, Veltri RW: Analysis of repeated biopsy results within 1 year after a noncancer diagnosis. Urology 2000, 55: 553–559.
[15] Zlotta AR, Schulman CC. Clinical evolution of prostatic intraepithelial neoplasia. Eur Urol. 1999, 35: 498-503.
[16] •JC Jr. Prostate biopsy strategies. Nat Clin Pract Urol. 2007, 4: 505-511. Detailed literature review of various published approaches to prostate biopsy schemes.
[17] Bostwick DG, Srigley J, Grignon D, et al.: Atypical adenomatous hyperplasia of the prostate: morphologic criteria for its distinction from well-differentiated carcinoma. Hum Pathol 24: 819–832.
[18] Rietbergen JBW, Boeken Kruger AE, Hoedemaeker RF, et al.: Repeat screening for prostate cancer after 1-year followup in 984 biopsied men: Clinical and pathological features of detected cancer. J. Urol. 1998, 160: 2121–2125.
[19] Chen ME, Troncoso P, Johnston D, Tang K, Babaian RJ: Prostate cancer detection: relationship to prostate size. Urology 1999, 53: 764–768.
[20] Remzi M, Djavan B, Wammack R, et al.: Can total and transition zone volume of the prostate determine whether to perform a repeat biopsy? Urology 2003, 61: 161–166.
[21] Basillote JB, Armenakas NA, Hochberg DA, Fracchia JA: Influence of prostate volume in the detection of prostate cancer. Urology 2003, 61: 167–171.
[22] Ung JO, San Francisco IF, Regan MM, DeWolf WC, Olumi AF: The relationship of prostate gland volume to extended needle biopsy on prostate cancer detection. J Urol 2003, 169: 130–135.
[23] Sajadi KP, Kim T, Terris MK, Brown JA, Lewis RW: High yield of saturation prostate biopsy for patients with previous negative biopsies and small prostates. Urology. 2007, 70: 691-695.
[24] Okada K, Kojima M, Naya Y, et al.: Correlation of histological inflammation in needle biopsy specimens with serum prostate-specific antigen levels in men with negative biopsy for prostate cancer. Urology 2000, 55: 892–898.
[25] Hasui Y, Marutsuka K, Asada Y, et al.: Relationship between serum prostate specific antigen and histological prostatitis in patients with benign prostatic hyperplasia. Prostate 1994, 25: 91–96.
[26] Nadler RB, Humphrey PA, Smith DS, Catalona WJ, Ratliff TL: Effect of inflammation and benign prostatic hyperplasia on elevated serum prostate specific antigen levels. J Urol 1995, 154: 407–413.
[27] Morote J, Lopez M, Encabo G, de Torres IM: Effect of inflammation and benign prostatic enlargement on total and percent free serum prostatic specific antigen. Eur Urol 2000, 37: 537–540.

[28] Abouassaly R, Tan N, Moussa A, Jones JS. Risk of prostate cancer after diagnosis of atypical glands suspicious for carcinoma on saturation and traditional biopsies. J Urol. 2008,180: 911-914.

[29] Davis M, Sofer M, Kim SS, Soloway MS: The procedure of transrectal ultrasound guided biopsy of the prostate: a survey of patient preparation and biopsy technique. J Urol. 2002, 167:566-70.

[30] Ochiai A, Babaian RJ: Update on prostate biopsy technique. Curr Opin Urol. 2004, 14: 157-162.

[31] Feliciano J, Teper E, Ferrandino M, Macchia RJ, Blank W, Grunberger I, Colon I. The incidence of fluoroquinolone resistant infections after prostate biopsy—are fluoroquinolones still effective prophylaxis? J Urol. 2008, 179: 952-955.

[32] Hong YM, Lai FC, Chon CH, McNeal JE, Presti JC Jr.: Impact of prior biopsy scheme on pathologic features of cancers detected on repeat biopsies. Urol Oncol. 2004, 22: 7-10.

[33] Kamoi K, Troncoso P, Babaian RJ: Strategy for repeat biopsy in patients with high grade prostatic intraepithelial neoplasia. J Urol. 2000, 163: 819-823.

[34] Shepherd D, Keetch DW, Humphrey PA, Smith DS, Stahl D: Repeat biopsy strategy in men with isolated prostatic intraepithelial neoplasia on prostate needle biopsy. J Urol. 1996, 156: 460-462.

[35] Patel AR, Jones JS, Zhou M, Schoenfield L, Magi-Galluzzi C. Parasagittal biopsies are more important as part of an initial biopsy strategy than as part of a repeat biopsy strategy: observations from a unique population. Prostate Cancer Prostatic Dis. 2007, 10: 352-355.

[36] Stamey TA: Making the most out of six systematic sextant biopsies. Urology 1995, 45: 2-12.

[37] Eskew LA, Bare RL, McCullough DL. Systematic 5 region prostate biopsy is superior to sextant method for diagnosing carcinoma of the prostate. J Urol. 1997, 157: 199-202.

[38] Presti JC Jr, Chang JJ, Bhargava V, Shinohara K: The optimal systematic prostate biopsy scheme should include 8 rather than 6 biopsies: results of a prospective clinical trial. J Urol 2000, 163: 163-166.

[39] Babaian RJ, Toi A, Kamoi K, et al.: A comparative analysis of sextant and an extended 11-core multisite directed biopsy strategy. J Urol. 2000, 163: 152-157.

[40] Mian BM, Naya Y, Okihara K, et al.: Predictors of cancer in repeat extended multisite prostate biopsy in men with previous negative extended multisite biopsy. Urology. 2002, 60:836-840.

[41] Terris MK, McNeal JE, Stamey TA: Transrectal ultrasound imaging and ultrasound guided prostate biopsies in the detection of residual carcinoma in clinical stage A carcinoma of the prostate. J Urol 1992, 146: 864-869.

[42] Liu IJ, Macy M, Lai YH, Terris MK: Critical evaluation of the current indications for transition zone biopsies. Urology 2001, 57: 1117-1120.

[43] Fleshner N, Klotz L. Role of "saturation biopsy" in the detection of prostate cancer among difficult diagnostic cases. Urology. 2002, 6: 93-97.

[44] Meng MV, Franks JH, Presti JC Jr, Shinohara K: The utility of apical anterior horn biopsies in prostate cancer detection. Urol Oncol 2003, 21: 361-365.

[45] Wright JL, Ellis WJ: Improved prostate cancer detection with anterior apical prostate biopsies. Urol Oncol. 2006, 24: 492-495.

[46] Stewart CS, Leibovich BC, Weaver AL, Lieber MM: Prostate cancer diagnosis using a saturation needle biopsy technique after previous negative sextant biopsies. J Urol. 2001, 166: 86-92.

[47] Jones JS, Patel A, Schoenfield L: Saturation technique does not improve cancer detection as an initial prostate biopsy strategy. J Urol. 2006, 175: 485-488.

[48] Ashley RA, Inman BA, Routh JC, Mynderse LA, Gettman MT, Blute ML. Reassessing the diagnostic yield of saturation biopsy of the prostate. Eur Urol. 2008, 53: 976-981.

[49] Igel TC, Knight MK, Young PR: Systematic transperineal ultrasound guided template biopsy of the prostate in patients at high risk. J Urol. 2001, 165: 1575-1579.

[50] Pinkstaff DM, Igel TC, Petrou SP, Broderick GA, Wehle MJ, Young PR. Systematic transperineal ultrasound-guided template biopsy of the prostate: three-year experience. Urology. 2005, 65: 735-739.

[51] G. Draisma, R. Boer and S.J. Otto *et al.*, Lead times and overdetection due to prostate-specific antigen screening: estimates from the European Randomized Study of Screening for Prostate Cancer, *J Natl Cancer Inst* 95 (2003), pp. 868–878.

[52] Meelan Bul, Roderick C.N. van den Bergh, Antti Rannikko, Riccardo Valdagni, Tom Pickles, Chris H. Bangma, Monique J. Roobol, Predictors of Unfavourable Repeat Biopsy Results in Men Participating in a Prospective Active Surveillance Program, European Urology, In Press, Corrected Proof, Available online 20 June 2011, ISSN 0302-2838, DOI: 10.1016/j.eururo.2011.06.027.

[53] Roderick C.N. van den Bergh, Stijn Roemeling, Monique J. Roobol, Tineke Wolters, Fritz H. Schroder, Chris H. Bangma, Prostate-Specific Antigen Kinetics in Clinical Decision-Making During Active Surveillance for Early Prostate Cancer--A Review, European Urology, Volume 54, Issue 3, September 2008, Pages 505-516, ISSN 0302-2838, DOI: 10.1016/j.eururo.2008.06.040.

[54] Matthew J. Resnick, Daniel J. Lee, Laurie Magerfleisch, Keith N. Vanarsdalen, John E. Tomaszewski, Alan J. Wein, S. Bruce Malkowicz, Thomas J. Guzzo, Repeat Prostate Biopsy and the Incremental Risk of Clinically Insignificant Prostate Cancer, Urology, Volume 77, Issue 3, March 2011, Pages 548-552, ISSN 0090-4295, DOI: 10.1016/j.urology.2010.08.063.

[55] Andrew J. Vickers, Tineke Wolters, Caroline J. Savage, Angel M. Cronin, M. Frank O'Brien, Monique J. Roobol, Gunnar Aus, Peter T. Scardino, Jonas Hugosson, Fritz H. Schroder, Hans Lilja, Prostate Specific Antigen Velocity Does Not Aid Prostate Cancer Detection in Men With Prior Negative Biopsy, The Journal of Urology, Volume 184, Issue 3, September 2010, Pages 907-912, ISSN 0022-5347, DOI: 10.1016/j.juro.2010.05.029.

[56] Zhou M, Magi-Galluzzi C. Clinicopathological features of prostate cancers detected after an initial diagnosis of 'atypical glands suspicious for cancer'. Pathology. 2010 Jun;42(4):334-8.

[57] Lee BH, Hernandez AV, Zaytoun O, Berglund RK, Gong MC, Jones JS. Utility of Percent Free Prostate-specific Antigen in Repeat Prostate Biopsy. Urology. 2011 Jun 16. [Epub ahead of print]

[58] Nam RK, Saskin R, Lee Y, Liu Y, Law C, Klotz LH, Loblaw DA, Trachtenberg J, Stanimirovic A, Simor AE, Seth A, Urbach DR, Narod SA. Increasing hospital admission rates for urological complications after transrectal ultrasound guided prostate biopsy. J Urol. 2010 Mar;183(3):963-8. Epub 2010 Jan 20.

[59] B. Djavan, M. Waldert, A. Zlotta, P. Dobronski, C. Seitz, M. Remzi *et al.*, Safety and morbidity of first and repeat transrectal ultrasound guided prostate needle biopsies: results of a prospective European prostate cancer detection study. *J. Urol.* 166 (2001), pp. 856–860.